TIME TO BLOSSOM

Harvesting Wellness and Wisdom on Your Personal Life Journey

Anne Marie Frizzell

BALBOA
PRESS
A DIVISION OF HAY HOUSE

Copyright © 2015 Anne Marie Frizzell.

All rights reserved. No part of this book may be used or reproduced by any means, graphic, electronic, or mechanical, including photocopying, recording, taping or by any information storage retrieval system without the written permission of the author except in the case of brief quotations embodied in critical articles and reviews.

Balboa Press books may be ordered through booksellers or by contacting:

Balboa Press
A Division of Hay House
1663 Liberty Drive
Bloomington, IN 47403
www.balboapress.com
1 (877) 407-4847

Because of the dynamic nature of the Internet, any web addresses or links contained in this book may have changed since publication and may no longer be valid. The views expressed in this work are solely those of the author and do not necessarily reflect the views of the publisher, and the publisher hereby disclaims any responsibility for them.

The author of this book does not dispense medical advice or prescribe the use of any technique as a form of treatment for physical, emotional, or medical problems without the advice of a physician, either directly or indirectly. The intent of the author is only to offer information of a general nature to help you in your quest for emotional and spiritual well-being. In the event you use any of the information in this book for yourself, which is your constitutional right, the author and the publisher assume no responsibility for your actions.

Any people depicted in stock imagery provided by Thinkstock are models, and such images are being used for illustrative purposes only.
Certain stock imagery © Thinkstock.

Print information available on the last page.

ISBN: 978-1-5043-4201-8 (sc)
ISBN: 978-1-5043-4200-1 (e)

Balboa Press rev. date: 12/03/2015

CONTENTS

FOREWORD xi

PREFACE xvii
    Time to Blossom xx

ACKNOWLEDGEMENT xxvii

INTRODUCTION xxix

PART ONE 1
Your Well Life Journey
    Wellness- A Journey of Discovery 1
    The Path to Personal Freedom 2

PART TWO 7
Family Matters
    The Wellness Nursery 7
    Guardians of Wellness 9
    Digging out the Roots 13
    Sowing and Growing Wellness 18

PART THREE 21
The Inner Commentator
    Your Personal Radio Station 21
    Licence to Broadcast 23
    Towards a New Script 26

PART FOUR 29
The Fountain of Truth-Cornerstones of Wellness
    Beyond the Mask... 29
    From a Place of Love 31
    Freedom through Gratitude..32
    Farewell Judge and Jury 35
    Getting to the Truth of the Matter 36

PART FIVE... 39
Turning Obstacles into Building Blocks
    Wellness beyond Grief... 39
    Who Put the Knot in Your Can?.. 42
    A Different Outlook... 44
    Eat Well to Feel Well 45
    Wellness in Motion 49
    Sleep Glorious Sleep.. 53
    The Steering Wheel of Your Life 55
    Releasing Stress and Restoring Balance.................................. 58
    From Busyness to Mindfulness..61
    A Daily Dose of Laughter.. 64
    The Working Well 65

PART SIX 70
Next Steps on Your Personal Life Journey
    Growing Your Personal Wellness Foundation 70
    From a Dream to a Vision 74
    From Vision to Reality 77

AFTERWORD 83

BIBLIOGRAPHY 87

ABOUT THE AUTHOR... 89

RESOURCES 91

For Erica-The lotus flower in the garden of my life.

"God, grant me the serenity to accept the things I cannot change, the courage to change the things I can and the wisdom to know the difference."

Reinhold Niebuhr

FOREWORD

The concept of wellness was influenced by the work of humanistic psychologists (e.g. Maslow, Rogers, Perls, Satir, etc.) who saw that actualizing human potential was a natural human process.

Over the years volumes have been written on ways to develop our potential and an equal collection of volumes about how to be well. While the human potential movement tended to stay centered in the world of intellect and emotion and often, by default, the world of psychotherapy, the budding wellness movement (which caught fire in the mid-seventies) expanded the nature of growth to include our whole lives, especially the physical and health aspects of our lives. When a person realises that their wellness, their summative state of health and wellbeing, is really about their own personal growth, the shifts in attitude, belief and behaviour truly usher in positive change.

Sadly, in the last decade or so, we have seen the burgeoning wellness field slip away from its holistic, personal growth/human potential roots and become fixated, all too often, on weight loss, smoking cessation and employee health driven by health-risk reduction models. In recent times the term "Wellbeing" has evolved as a way to remind us to return to a concept of whole-person wellness and embrace mind, body, spirit and environment. A return to our holistic roots seems in order.

Anne Marie Frizzell's work is about reminding people that they are whole people, and to remember that wellness/wellbeing is, at the bottom line, about personal growth. I've often said to the thousands of health and wellness coaches we have trained worldwide, that a coach's job is to remind people that they have choices. Yet as Anne Marie shows us in this book, life is not quite as sweet and simple as "choose to be well."

Anne Marie, in reference to dis-ease, addiction and recovery brings out a reminder of the healing that sometimes needs to precede the process of developing and implementing a wellness plan. Sometimes our Personal Life Journey begins with lightening our backpack of some of the stones that we have been carrying far too long.

Before my shift into the world of life coaching and helping develop the field of wellness coaching I worked as a doctoral level psychologist for many years. I saw how effective people could be at healing old wounds of the past, at clearing out self-defeating ways of thinking and behaving through the hard work of personal therapy. People learn and grow and heal in many ways. An outdoor adventure experience, or reconnection and reconciliation with a family member might provide profound healing for one, yet another person may need the safety and support of more serious psychotherapeutic treatment. Coaching was never designed to handle the remedial treatment that some clients may need. Effective, professional coaches are trained to recognise their scope of competency and to facilitate referral to licensed mental health professionals when appropriate.

The need for an ally to help in overcoming one's internal and external barriers to change will never go away. While there is a place for simplistic computer-generated reminder programs that nudge people to exercise often, make the best food choices, etc., the need for a real, live ally to talk with about what gets in the way of success is a significant reason for the rise in popularity of wellness and health coaching. External barriers can often be addressed with support, effective strategizing, and experimenting with new behaviours. Internal barriers, however, are often the tougher nut to crack because it means work on the inside...the inside of us.

Perhaps our most challenging internal barriers are the attitudes and beliefs that we adhere most strongly to, yet are the least aware of. It is so easy for a person to develop a view of the world that is very self-defeating, yet be blind to how it holds them back. A self-fulfilling prophecy can be in play when a cynical view of the world distorts perception of events as negative and the person sees how justified they were to be cynical about things to start with! There is abundant literature that pessimists have worse health statistics than optimists. The exciting new work in Positive Psychology confirms that those who hold a more positive ratio in their view of life events and experiences have better health and wellbeing. Yet as Anne Marie reminds us, there is more to our own inner work than just waking up one morning looking in the mirror and saying "You're terrific!"

Emotions are part of life and everyone on a growth path will find them surfacing, and that is a good thing. Personal growth that does not include our emotional selves is usually temporary. Coaches do, indeed, help their clients to deal with feelings. Process coaching, as it is called, is a key skill in the repertoire of a well-trained coach. The approach emphasises facilitating the work that the client does with their emotions, rather than some sort of treatment approach.

One method that coaches find helpful with their clients as they grow is working with the "Inner Critic", also known as "The Gremlin", or as Anne Marie brilliantly refers to it; "The Inner Commentator." Ironically one of the times we are most vulnerable to the words of this doubting part of ourselves is right when we are making progress on our growth path. Our success threatens the status quo and seems to trigger our fears, doubts and all of these nay-saying recordings in our heads. Listen to them and they will grow louder. Tune out of that radio station (as Anne Marie puts it) and their power is lost.

Personal growth, making our way towards living our Well Life Vision, is not always about barriers and troubling psychological challenges. For all of us there is a point where, in order to grow, we have to take stock of ourselves and our wellness, create a vision of the life we truly want to live and identify the gap between where we are and where we want to be. What has to change for us to get there becomes our wellness plan or map. Then comes the gritty work of executing that plan, and achieving the support to sustain it for the rest of our entire lives. Insight is not enough. Vision is not enough. It is a commitment to living our lives differently for the remainder of our days here on the planet.

What Anne Marie Frizzell includes in this book is the remaining piece of the life-change puzzle; how to get there. I sometimes speak about "Getting Behavioural About Being Holistic". We must wisely review our lives through a holistic lens and take it all in like we are floating in a hot-air balloon, able to see from horizon to horizon. Then, to make lasting lifestyle change, we must come back down to earth, go sit at a table with our sleeves rolled up, and draw up a map of specifically, behaviourally, how we will proceed on our journey towards the destination we want. Anne Marie draws upon her wellness coaching training and shares much of the key ingredients of the Real Balance Wellness Mapping 360° Methodology™ for how to do exactly this. This methodology has been taught to thousands of health and wellness coaches around the globe and is often cited by our students as the most valuable process that they have ever been taught about how to assist someone in succeeding at lasting lifestyle improvement.

Abraham Maslow often spoke about self-actualization compared to self-image actualization. He distinguished how actualizing our potential was not about achieving this notion of who we should be, but to continually be in the process of becoming who we truly are. The health and wellness field today is replete with admonitions to be a certain way, look a certain way, and of course, get there by buying a certain product. In coaching, and in this book, we counter with a process of finding and bringing forward our true selves. When coaching is at its highest level it is transformative. When a client says "I'm a whole new person now!" they are not really saying that they have become someone else. They are revealing the incredible person they are at their beautiful core. Now, they are living who they are.

>Michael Arloski, Ph.D., PCC, CWP
>CEO and Founder of Real Balance Global Wellness Services, Inc.
>Board member of The National Wellness Institute. Founding member of the executive team of The National Consortium for Credentialing Health and Wellness Coaches. Author of *Wellness Coaching for Lasting Lifestyle Change*, (2007, 2nd Ed. 2009)

PREFACE

Everyone is on a personal life journey involving a quest to discover and fulfil their life purpose and in doing so to live a satisfying and happy life. The pursuit of happiness, success or personal fulfilment is at times impeded by futile attempts to control life events, instead of recognising the difference between that which cannot be controlled, and that which one has the personal power to change. Often in the pursuit of happiness and success the true purpose and meaning of life is missed. Primarily because energies are focussed on human "doing" instead of human "being". In the search for a *better life* many overlook the magnificence of the life they already have and as a result, fulfilment and happiness seem out of reach.

For many people life involves working hard and/or pursuing further education or training to improve their knowledge, skills and career opportunities. When not working or studying they may participate in family activities, hobbies or became involved with their local community. They lead busy lives yet for many, life feels out of balance and they sense that something is missing. It can take some tough life lessons for them to realise that they do not have a well life balance because they are completely focussed on "doing" instead of "being." They do not appreciate that the power to find balance, peace of mind and live a well and happy life rests primarily with them and does not come from some external source.

Throughout our life we are presented with challenging lessons veiled in either positive or negative life experiences. Central to living well and wisely is being open to the lessons life offers you, focussing on the areas of your life where you can make changes and accepting or letting go of that which you cannot change or control.

My career brought me initially into nursing and for many years I had the privilege of working in rehabilitation training and occupational support services for adults with disabilities. During this time I began to establish the foundations for my future work in wellness and health coaching. For a person with a disability to achieve positive outcomes, the education, training or occupation they participate in must be meaningful and centred on their personal interests, abilities and aspirations. The same principle applies to each of our lives. To fulfil our potential and experience personal life satisfaction we need to focus on our interests, our abilities and our dreams, and then, do what is necessary to make them a priority in how we live our lives.

Over the years I also had the opportunity to engage with individuals who had experience of living with addiction. These individuals helped me understand the impact of dis-ease and addiction on their quality of life and personal wellness. They taught me that healing and recovery is individual and encompasses wellness of the mind, the body and the spirit. It is strengthened by reaching out to and connecting with others for support. To be truly well we have to care for and nurture our mind, our body and our spirit and this realisation ignited my interest in a whole person approach to wellness.

As I awakened to the significance of a well mind, body and spirit I discovered that many people are completely missing the point of life. By constantly looking to the future and trying to predict what is to come or, by trying to control outcomes, we miss out on the most important time of our lives which is the present moment in which we exist. There is only this moment and it will never be relived so make sure you live it well! You should draw comfort from knowing that the here and now is the most important point on your life journey and you do not have to expend valuable mental energy worrying about what may or may not happen in the future. By giving full focus to what you are doing in each moment, your life will have meaning and you will know your primary purpose at all times.

The more immersed I became in wellness as a way of life it became obvious that a person centred approach to wellness is essential if we are to support people to build the bridge between wellness of their mind, their body and their spirit. I began exploring wellness models and this led me to wellness and health coaching and the work of, among others, Dr Michael Arloski, Ph.D, Real Balance Global Wellness Services. I was delighted when Dr Arloski brought his wellness and health coach training to Ireland in 2012. When I embarked on this training I embraced the similarities between the principles of the Real Balance Wellness Mapping 360° Methodology™ developed by Dr Arloski (2007) and the research I had conducted in relation to quality of life and person centred planning for persons with disabilities.

Life satisfaction is not derived solely from social, occupational, educational or material achievements but rather by the extent to which you acknowledge your inner truth and honour that truth in the way you live your life. I hold firmly to the belief that life satisfaction is personal, and our individual quest for wellness of our mind, body and spirit will inform our life choices, our lifestyle behaviours and ultimately our personal wellness foundation. Wellness and health coaching has given me a framework to apply these principle to my own life and to support others to do the same. Dr Arloski has kindly granted permission to incorporate aspects of the Real Balance Wellness Mapping 360° Methodology™ in this book and for that I am deeply grateful.

If we accept that each of us is on a personal life journey then every day is an opportunity to cultivate wellness and wisdom, discover our inner truth and live in alignment with that truth. Before we begin our journey through this book I want to share with you a short story about personal discovery and wisdom.

Time to Blossom

Once upon a time in a distant kingdom lived a radiant being called Sutol. Sutol glowed brightly, exuded happiness and had a blissful existence. One day Sutol noticed that some of the radiant beings were disappearing and then reappearing again at a later time. When the radiant beings reappeared they seemed to glow brighter than before they had left. Sutol wondered what was going on so the next time one of the radiant beings reappeared he asked him where he had been. The radiant being told Sutol that he had been on a special personal journey and had now returned home. Sutol wanted to know all about this journey but the radiant being would only say "be patient, enjoy the present moment, and when you are ready you too will go on your personal journey."

Sutol was not satisfied with this response and set about asking other radiant beings about their journey. Each said the same thing, "be patient, enjoy the present moment, and when you are ready you too will go on your personal journey." Sutol was becoming impatient with their responses so he went to see Harmony one of the wise leaders of the land to find out what was going on. Harmony was expecting Sutol because at some point all radiant beings will begin to sense that there is more to be learned and will become thirsty for knowledge. The only way they can acquire this knowledge is to embark on a personal journey of discovery. It would soon be time for Sutol to embark on his journey.

Harmony explained to Sutol that each radiant being is perfect just as they are but, to evolve and become a wise leader they must harvest wellness and wisdom and learn to live in alignment with their inner truth. Harmony explained that there is a fountain of truth and wisdom within each radiant being but because they exist in a land where love, joy and serenity are their only experiences, they are not challenged to access this fountain of truth and wisdom. When a radiant being unlocks the fountain of truth and wisdom inside themselves they are capable of becoming a wise leader. Sutol was thirsty for truth and wisdom so he pleaded with Harmony to teach him what he needed to know to become a wise leader.

Harmony explained to Sutol that to access truth and wisdom he would have to undertake a series of lessons which are presented during your personal journey. Harmony compared a personal journey to a quest to find hidden treasures which in Sutol's case were inner truth, wisdom and wellness. Harmony explained that each radiant being must attend LJ prep school to prepare for the journey.

On his personal journey Sutol would face many challenges and each would offer a lesson that would bring Sutol closer to inner truth, wisdom and wellness. Some of the lessons would be difficult and Sutol would at times experience pain and sadness but at other times there would be much love and happiness. Even though this journey sounded demanding Sutol was thirsty for wisdom and knowledge and so enrolled in LJ prep school. LJ prep school stands for Life Journey preparation school and Sutol was its newest student.

Harmony informed Sutol that the personal journey to be undertaken is called living and that Sutol would go to live on a wonderful planet called earth for an agreed period of time. While on earth Sutol would become a human being and would live there alongside other human beings. When his life journey is complete Sutol would return home ready to take his place as a wise leader. Harmony explained to Sutol that his purpose on earth would be to experience a series of life lessons and as each one is learned Sutol would access the fountain of wisdom and his inner truth would be revealed.

Harmony explained that the radiant beings in this majestic land emit love and happiness because they are spirits and each spirit is unique, pure and perfect. Harmony taught Sutol that his spirit is also unique, pure and perfect and is reflective of his inner truth. Therefore he must remain true to his spirit at all times. Harmony informed Sutol that as a human being he would have free will to choose how he responded when faced with each life experience. The choice would be his whether or not to embrace the lesson offered in each experience. The choices Sutol makes, explained Harmony, will determine how aligned he is to his inner truth and how much wisdom he acquires.

Harmony explained that as a human being Sutol would have a physical body which would be the vessel to carry his spirit during his time on earth. Sutol was instructed to feed his physical body with healthy food, hydrate it with water, exercise it regularly and ensure it has adequate rest and sleep. One of the responsibilities as a human being, explained Harmony, is to accept, love and care for your body regardless of what it looks like. Each human being has a physical body specially designed for their unique spirit so there is a perfect match regardless of what the body looks like. It made sense to Sutol that if you have been given a specially designed body to carry you on your life journey you should treat it well.

A large part of the preparation for his life journey was learning about the mind and thoughts. Harmony explained that not only would there be a physical body there would also be a thing called a mind-body which produces thoughts, emotions and feelings which in turn influence your choices and behaviour. Sutol was instructed to develop a conscious awareness of his thoughts and to recognise those that could undermine the wellness of his mind or body or draw him away from his inner truth. Harmony explained that often times human beings give power to negative thoughts and this can lead to harmful behaviour patterns that prevent them from fulfilling their divine life purpose.

Harmony provided guidance to Sutol on how to live alongside other human beings and explained that the starting point would be learning to live with a family. Sutol's first teachers on his life journey would be his family and some of the lessons they offer him would be pleasant but others may be complex or challenging. Harmony went onto explain to Sutol about relationships, school, work, community, illness, money, science, media, recreation, war, the environment and the many other experiences and events human beings are exposed to, or create throughout their lifetime. He explained that in each experience there will be a lesson that will bring him a step closer to harvesting wellness and wisdom.

The duration of each human beings life journey is determined by the range of lessons they are required to learn. Some life journeys are long, others are short. The key explained Harmony, is to embrace each living day, seek only the truth and take good care of your precious mind, body and spirit. Once all his required life lessons are learned Sutol would be called home.

Sutol was an excellent student and was soon ready to embark on his personal life journey. Harmony informed Sutol that when he becomes human he will not remember this majestic land but that his spirit would remain within him while living on earth. Harmony emphasised the importance of Sutol attuning to his inner spirit and being guided by it throughout his life. His spirit and the guidance he has received in LJ prep school would be his blue print for living well. Harmony also explained that when he becomes human his parents will choose a special name for him and this will be his identify while living on earth. Sutol bid farewell to Harmony and commenced his quest for inner truth, wisdom and wellness. At that exact moment a new life was conceived and another personal life journey began.

When Sutol's life journey was complete he was welcomed home by Harmony who asked him to share what he had learned while living on planet earth. Sutol took a few moments to reflect on his experience and then gave this reply.

"It was an amazing journey with much joy but also some pain and sadness along the way. I met wonderful people who taught me about living well and enjoying life. They guided me to look within myself to find the answers to the questions I was presented with throughout my life. I also met some people who hurt me. At times I felt anger and resentment toward them and the longer I felt like this the more negative my thoughts became.

At one point in my life I felt like my mind was in a dark place and I wanted to quit this journey. While in this dark place I did not look after my physical body and I allowed negative thoughts to take control of my mind. It was like an ongoing commentary in my head spoken by an angry person. This voice kept telling me I was worthless and that other people did not like me. It also told me that I was a failure and that I deserved the hurt and pain I had experienced. I believed this commentary and at times I sought comfort in food, drugs, alcohol or other unhealthy activities. I stopped taking regular exercise and began to isolate myself from other people including some of my family. Because I believed that no one wanted to be around me I felt it was best to avoid the company of others as much as possible.

After a time in this dark place I began to feel lonely, my mind was in state of dis-ease and my body was becoming unwell. I realised that I had turned each painful life experience into a stumbling block and now I was on fragile ground. Although I was surviving I was not really living. I was thirsty for wellness and wanted to experience a feeling of joy and love in my life again. With a lot of effort I pulled myself out of this dark place and committed to cultivating wellness of my mind, my body and my spirit, tuning into my inner truth and fulfilling my life purpose.

Gradually and over time I began to rebuild my personal wellness foundation. I reached out for support from other people. Through them I began to realise that I had surrendered my free will to the voice of the negative inner commentator and had chosen anger and resentment over love and gratitude. At that moment I made a conscious decision to let go of anger which I realised was driven by fear, and to seek only love and truth. I began to accept that each person I met was also on a personal life journey and many were struggling just as I was. Once I accepted this I stopped judging others and gradually began to return to a state of wellness and inner peace. I fell in love with life and learned to accept myself just as I was, perfect despite my human imperfections.

My spirit was re-awakened to the wonderful gift that was my life, including the people I shared it with and the magnificent planet where I was blessed to live. I took responsibility for my life and strived to do my best in my relationships and daily activities. I embraced the education and occupation opportunities that were available to me. I began to take care of my body and I committed to protecting the environment for future generations. Even though I had damaged my physical body it had not let me down nor had it given up on me. I adopted a healthy diet, listened to and rested my body when it was tired and learned how to manage the stress in my life. I started to express gratitude for the good things and people in my life and I began to practice forgiveness.

I came to realise that I did not have to achieve perfection but just had to do my best. I acknowledged that I was responsible for my own behaviour, thoughts and actions and not those of other people. Once I accepted this it was as though a weight had lifted from my shoulders and I felt free. That was a turning point in how I lived my life from then onwards. I faced many challenges on my personal life journey but by accepting myself and others just as we are and striving for wellness of my mind, body and spirit, I began to enjoy life, and I found inner peace and a well life balance. I believe" said Sutol "that each of my life experiences was a step toward wellness, wisdom and discovering my inner truth. I know now that this was the ultimate purpose of my life."

Harmony was silent for a few moments, then smiled at Sutol and said, "Congratulations, you have blossomed into a wise leader who seeks and speaks only the truth. You will no longer be called Sutol. From this moment onwards you will be called Lotus." Today in the garden of life Lotus continues to blossom in wellness, wisdom and truth.

This is your time to blossom! Let's get started on building your personal wellness foundation, unlocking your inner truth, and harvesting wellness and wisdom so that you too can fulfil your divine life purpose.

ACKNOWLEDGEMENT

I would like to gratefully acknowledge my family and friends for the lessons and support on my personal life journey.

I wish to acknowledge each person who has experienced physical, mental or emotional ill health. You are all wellness warriors. I salute your courage and pray that you will blossom in wellness, reclaim your personal power and find peace and serenity in your lives.

I would like to extend my heartfelt thanks to Susan, Kathleen, Ann, Breda and Dan for challenging the status quo and remaining person centred in how they worked.

I would like to acknowledge every person with a disability whom I have worked with. Thank you for teaching me the importance of seeing beyond disabling barriers and maintaining a focus on what can be achieved in life.

I would like to extend my deep appreciation to Asha for guiding and supporting me on my spiritual journey.

I would like to thank Dr Michael Arloski for introducing me to wellness and health coaching, for encouraging me to live in accordance with my well life vision and for his inspiring work in promoting global wellness.

I wish to convey eternal gratitude to Imelda, Sylvia, Rose, Audrey, Tish, Mary C and Mary McG for the priceless gift of your wisdom and friendship.

INTRODUCTION

Dear Reader

This book has come about from my wish to share with you some of the pearls of wisdom and wellness I have discovered on my personal life journey. I do not claim to be a wellness expert but I hope that as you read this book you will be encouraged to make life choices that strengthen the foundations for wellness of your mind, your body and your spirit.

This book is designed to help you discover your inner truth, draw from the fountain of wisdom inside yourself and in doing so achieve a well life balance. It is divided into six parts which can be read in order or, if you prefer, start with the section you are most drawn to. Take time to absorb what is written and at your own pace start to apply some of the guidance offered.

Life takes each of us on an amazing personal journey, during which we are taught valuable lessons that move us toward achieving our full potential and blossoming into the person we are destined to become. The key to wellness is to enjoy the journey, harness wisdom and truth and embrace every living moment. When you have completed your life journey my wish for you is that you will have lived it well, achieved inner peace, experienced and shared much love and blossomed in wellness and wisdom.

Enjoy the journey!

PART ONE
Your Well Life Journey

Wellness- A Journey of Discovery

Most people at some point, start to wonder about the meaning and purpose of their life. When this happens it is the beginning of the quest to find inner truth, wisdom and wellness. It is the re-awakening of the spirit and is the point on your life journey when you are truly ready to harvest wellness of your mind, body and spirit.

Wellness means different things to different people and is informed by each individual's life experiences, their attitude, their personal values and their core beliefs. Wellness encompasses mind, body and spirit, and is influenced by what is going on in your life at this moment in time. Wellness of the body is linked to physical health, wellness of the mind is influenced by your mental or emotional state and spiritual wellness is underpinned by your belief system and the extent to which you live in alignment with these beliefs. If we broaden the concept further we recognise that whole person wellness is impacted by our physical and mental health, our relationships, our environment, our education, our occupation, our material wealth, our experience of stress, our social supports, the level of engagement we have with our community, our faith based or spiritual beliefs, and our ability to connect with our inner truth and to live by that truth. It is impossible therefore to talk about wellness without considering how all aspects of one's life will impact on it.

A key factor in how you perceive wellness is the mindset you adopt as you journey through life. A person may be going through treatment for cancer but may feel well today because their pain is under control. Someone else may have lost a family member but feels well because they are grateful for the memorable times spent with the person. Someone else may have a stressful job or may be struggling financially but feels well today because they have taken steps toward changing jobs or improving their finances. Someone else may be faced with a major life event but feels okay, because they trust that the God of their understanding will guide them to make the right decision or choices. Wellness therefore is significantly influenced by your perspective on life and the attitude you choose to adopt.

The human mind and body when it is functioning according to its genius design is at ease. When the harmony of our mind, body or spirit is disturbed we move away from wellness and toward dis-ease and illness. Dis-ease is the adversary of wellness so it is vital to strengthen your wellness foundation. Many people struggle to achieve balance in their lives because they are conflicted between their current lifestyle and what they instinctively know would be a better way of living. Regardless of the cause of this imbalance they struggle to make the changes that will move them toward increased life satisfaction and better wellness and health. By choosing not to make life changes they suppress their inner truth, surrender their personal power and continue to maintain low levels of wellness.

However when a person makes the decision to start living their life in accordance with their inner truth, they reclaim their personal power, honour their right to happiness and begin living in a meaningful way and with purpose. This marks the beginning of their personal wellness journey.

The Path to Personal Freedom

You are exactly where you are meant to be right now on your personal life journey. Your journey began when you were born and will continue until you die, and the time in between is what you are required to live. Many people spend a considerable amount of time focusing on their past or trying to predict or control their future. This "past to the future" thinking can get in the way of living well in the present moment. Present moment awareness is in essence, your *gateway to personal freedom*. The past is gone and the road ahead is yet to be travelled, so embrace this present moment and give your full attention to what you are doing right now, because this is your primary purpose.

Embracing the present moment requires you to become mindful and this can be challenging for many of the human race. It is not surprising that we are called a race since we are constantly rushing to meet some deadline or other. With this constant rushing and unrealistic pressures we put ourselves under we become exhausted, overwhelmed and start to burnout. We lose all sense of direction and become part of the so called *rat race*. If you stop to reflect on what you are actually achieving by speeding your way through life, you may well discover that the loss in terms of quality of life far outweighs the gains. The next time you feel hurried, stressed or under pressure to meet a deadline, take a moment to ask yourself "what am I gaining from this?" By asking this simple question you start to introduce mindfulness into your life and this will allow you to reflect on how meaningful and satisfying your life actually is.

Your early environment plays a significant part in setting the foundation for your future health and wellness. Parents play a central role in determining the social, emotional, physical, material and spiritual environment in the home which in turn influences the state of wellness experienced by the family. If a group of parents were asked about their vision for their child's future most would want their child to be healthy, happy and to achieve their full potential. Health, happiness and fulfilling ones potential are aspirations most people would also want for themselves. Take some time to consider what your vision is for your child's future or the future of a child you love. Consider what you would include if you had to create a plan to help the child achieve this vision.

Perhaps this plan may include a safe and secure physical environment, a loving family, a healthy diet, clean drinking water, regular exercise, adequate rest and sleep, protection from aggression, harm, neglect or abuse, high quality child care, access to excellent health care, a holistic education, a welcoming and supportive community, a wide range of social and recreation activities, a loyal circle of friends, enough material resources to live comfortably and perhaps some faith based activities aligned to your personal belief systems.

The path of life is not meant to be travelled alone so consider now who needs to be there to support the child on their life journey. This list may include parents and family, friends, teachers, neighbours, perhaps members of a faith community, career guidance counsellors, employers, coaches, volunteers, people who work in public services, retail, health care, education and so on. It is evident from this list that no child or indeed any adult can undertake their personal life journey without connecting with a variety of people and supports at different stages throughout their life.

The majority of people seek happiness and want this for their children but what does happiness mean and how can you create the conditions for happiness for yourself or your child? A child may be happy when they get a new toy or a treat but this is not true happiness. Rather it offers a temporary sense of satisfaction or enjoyment. The child feels happy because their material desires or expectations were met at that moment in time. However this is a short lived experience and to maintain that feeling the child would need to continuously receive toys or treats. Happiness is an internal experience and material goods will never create happiness. Undoubtedly they might bring comfort and pleasure and this may contribute to your sense of happiness, however material possessions in themselves do not make a person happy.

Each of you will be able to describe what happiness means to you and the older you become the less likely you are to equate happiness with material possessions. Happiness is underpinned by owning the freedom to accept and express who you really are. It involves choosing to live life according to your values, beliefs and dreams. It comes from knowing your inner truth and standing tall in that truth every day of your life, even when others do not agree with you. If you take away a person's freedom to express who they are, or judge them for being different, they may repress their inner truth and spend their life trying to impress, or be accepted by others. This results in a denial of self and can lead to physical, mental or spiritual pain and a loss of inner peace.

Society demands a level of conformity and imposes rules and regulations that direct people how to behave and in some cases how to think. When people deviate from these rules and regulations they may be viewed as rebellious or disloyal, and the focus of society then moves to re-establishing compliance. Many of these rules help maintain stability and social order but when rules inhibit freedom of expression and denial of one's inner truth then people begin to move away from wellness toward dis-ease and dissatisfaction.

Imagine for a moment how you would feel if you had to hide who you really are because you were afraid you would be discriminated against, shunned, criticised or rejected by others. This can apply to anyone and some readers may have had this experience as a child or adult. If a child or adult is discouraged from being true to whom she or he really is or their freedom of expression is denied, they will become unhappy. If they are constantly being compared to others and criticised for what they say or do, they quickly learn that to please others and gain acceptance they must behave in a certain way. In doing so they may suppress their feelings or fail to honour and give expression to their values and inner beliefs. This does not make for a happy childhood or adulthood and represents a denial of oneself and ones truth.

Happiness can flourish through self expression and by living in alignment with your inner truth. However if self expression is inhibited, the inner radiance of the person will not shine through. To blossom in wellness and wisdom we must nurture our own inner truth and that of our children. Only then, can meaningful world order be achieved, whereby each person reclaims their personal freedom and blossoms in wellness, love and happiness.

PART TWO
Family Matters

The Wellness Nursery

Some people hold a belief that each person has a soul that enters into a life contract before they are born, as in the earlier story about Sutol. They believe that this contract sets out the range of lessons the person must learn in order to fulfil their true potential and divine life purpose. The soul, it is believed, chooses the family that will provide the experiences and lessons it needs to flourish as a human being. Many would argue against this belief on the basis that they would not have chosen their particular family had they been given a choice. Whether this belief is true or not is largely irrelevant but what remains true is that your family teaches you valuable life lessons, even if at times you do not like the experience or want to resist the lessons on offer. It is through these lessons that the fountain of wisdom and truth inside of you is gradually revealed.

There is a societal expectation that you will love, honour and be loyal to your family at all times. This expectation may be hard to endorse, if your family has not been supportive or loving toward you or each other in the past. If someone in your family has hurt you deeply it can seem too big a challenge to love and honour them. By not doing so you may be viewed as disloyal and this may cause you to doubt your own judgement and beliefs. When you start to question your personal judgement or beliefs this begins to impact on your self efficacy and your ability to form trusting relationships.

The family is your first school of socialisation and it is here that the seeds of wellness and wisdom are sown. Families by their nature tend to create a cocoon for the protection and maintenance of the family unit. Preserving unity sometimes takes precedence over the needs of individual family members. Often there is an unwritten code of behaviour that governs conduct within the family.

This code of conduct provides the etiquette to be observed when families are in each other's company or when representing the family to the outside world. Each member learns from experience how to avoid stepping on interpersonal landmines or triggering arguments or disputes within the family. The experience of family, although at times challenging, teaches you how to navigate your life journey.

Within family you learn how to communicate, to take turns, to ask for your needs to be met, to share, to help each other, to work as a team, to stand up for yourself, to assert your personality and to voice your opinion. Family also reflects community in that its members have to work collaboratively so that everyone benefits from the shared effort. If family members find common ground on which to work together then each member will have their needs met and will be capable of forming meaningful relationships with people outside of the family and in the wider community. If you are encouraged to voice your opinion within the family you will feel valued. This sense of being valued provides nourishment for your wellness foundation and strengthens your capacity to blossom in wellness and wisdom as an adult.

The physical, mental and spiritual wellness of each member of the family is important as is the collective wellness of the family as a unit. The extension of family is the local community and the extension of local community is the global community. If we nurture wellness at a personal level we can cultivate wellness at family level which in turn will foster wellness at community level. Communities of wellness can have a powerful impact on global wellness, hence the importance of building the foundations for wellness at every opportunity. As a member of a family you are personally responsible for growing your own wellness foundation and unless you cultivate your own wellness you will not be equipped to influence wellness within your family, your community or the wider world. It may seem like a big responsibility for one person but each of us has the capability to positively influence the energy and life force of our planet every day. We do so by being a role model for personal wellness and by practicing acceptance and forgiveness within our family and with those we meet on our life journey.

Guardians of Wellness

Your life is an unconventional teacher as it gives you the test first and the lessons afterwards. Parents play a key role in determining the extent to which a child develops a strong foundation for wellness and self esteem. For a child to blossom in wellness and wisdom they require nurturing and guidance from parents who are tending to their own wellness foundation. To do so, parents must mind what matters in their life and the life of their child. Being a parent is one of the toughest roles people undertake and when it is being balanced with work and other commitments it can be exceptionally difficult to focus on wellness and to be mindful. Mindfulness can help diffuse a potentially volatile situation with a child or another family member but it requires regular practice for it to become a way of parenting.

If you are a parent, the next time you are faced with a difficult situation with your child stop, take a deep breath and ask yourself "what would be most helpful right at this moment?" Your inner voice may be pressuring you to shout out or lose your temper, but before you react consider how helpful such a response would be and what alternative approach you could adopt. Your answer may not fully extinguish your frustration or anger but it will give you time to turn down the volume of the negative inner voice and allow the voice of common sense to speak instead. You do not have to like a particular situation but igniting it or adding fuel to it only causes further hurt or pain.

In many families parents are genuinely eager to hear what their child has learned at kindergarten, nursery, pre-school or school and get excited about the smallest of achievements. If the parent is practicing mindfulness and has established their own wellness foundation they will freely praise the child and encourage them to continue with their efforts. However some parents who have not cultivated their own wellness foundation may show little interest in their child's learning or may find it difficult to praise their child for their achievements. Some may even dismiss their child's work or may be too busy to give attention to it.

Nowadays people live extraordinarily busy lives and because many parents feel under constant time pressure, mindfulness may not be high on their agenda. Often they have limited time to give undivided attention to their child. The child may be keen to show the parent their work but the parent may dismiss the child by telling them they will look at it later or that they are too busy.

The intent of the parent is not to hurt the child's feelings but, if this becomes a pattern the child quickly learns not to bother mum or dad. The child may over time, develop the belief that their work has little or no value and some may extend this belief to their own self worth. If this limiting belief becomes embedded it will erode the childs self esteem and self efficacy.

Parents or family members sometimes give conflicting messages to children in terms of what they say or by their behaviour. Some conflicting messages children receive include; a parent showing love and then suddenly withdrawing it, offering praise yet being quick to criticise, setting rules for children yet breaking these rules themselves, demanding respectful behaviour from the child yet acting disrespectfully toward others, shouting at the child yet telling the child to stop shouting, telling the child they are too busy to play as they sit in front of the television, telling the child to go out and exercise yet never bringing the child for a walk, telling the child to go to bed early yet sitting up late surfing the internet or watching television, telling the child to say their prayers yet never praying with their child or, telling the child to grow up when the child is still a child. The more you practice mindfulness the less likely you are to give conflicting messages to your child.

Every day in the life of a parent is like an experimental study whereby they try out different approaches to parenting and discover that what works today may not work tomorrow. They learn "on the job" so to speak and they become wise about parenting with the benefit of hindsight. This may be the reason why many grandparents are keen to offer parenting advice to their own adult children. They have been there, and have learned many parenting lessons along the way. However each child is unique and one size or type of parenting does not fit all children. Knowledge is helpful and advice maybe freely offered by others, but ultimately parenting is personal and no two children are the same.

If a parent views their role as that of educator, guide and supporter they can use difficult situations to teach their child about relationships and conflict. When this approach is adopted the family becomes a place where fundamental life lessons are imparted and the seeds of wisdom and respect are planted in the mind of the child. The earlier children experience these life lessons the more wisdom they will absorb as they journey through the University of Life.

Each child has a unique personality and often struggle to express themselves and be heard in a world that demands conformity. Some parents automatically reprimand their own child if they get into dispute with another child, instead of establishing the facts first. This can happen in families where the parents themselves were not respected as a child, or were treated unjustly. Perhaps they grew up in a culture where children had no right to voice their opinions, particularly if these were at odds with other adults including their parents.

Sadly some parents are likely to repeat the pattern they experienced and pass on negative and potentially destructive messages to their own children. When a child is blamed in the wrong they feel betrayed by the parent and emotionally wounded. Many people who experience harsh childhoods and who receive little love or respect, lose trust in adults and their self esteem becomes eroded. Thankfully however if they are treated with respect and given encouragement by adults later in life they can learn to trust again, their self esteem can be strengthened and their emotional wounds will heal. The good news for all parents is that each new day offers the opportunity to start again, learn from the past, honour your child's uniqueness and build your own wellness foundation.

The teenage years are when the seeds of wellness begin to germinate. Some children progress through adolescence and into young adulthood with relative ease but for others it can be a turbulent time. One day they are living through an emotional hurricane and the next day calm has been restored. The next hurricane may be only a few minutes, hours or days away but it is likely to return. Now throw a stressed parent into the equation and you have a perfect storm. The family can feel like a ship in stormy seas with the crew (the children including teenagers) looking for the captain (parents) to steer them to safety. If parents are stressed or feeling anxious about losing control it can be a challenging voyage. The more the captain tries to steer the ship back on course the more the crew resist and mutiny breaks out. Mainly because the crew are fearful of the unknown and feel the people whom they should be able to rely on are not keeping them safe. Surely the captain is supposed to know what they are doing and their job is to get the ship and crew safely home. The problem is that the map of life is only uncovered one point at a time so the voyage is often into uncharted waters. We have a general idea which direction we are going in life but there is no certainty about what lies ahead hence families have to figure it out one step at a time.

The teenager is also going through significant physiological changes which impact on their psychological and emotional wellbeing. This can be a frightening time where they feel they have little control over what is happening to them. Some teenagers experience little or no turbulence during the transition between childhood and adulthood but some parents struggle at this time to accept that their child is growing into an adult who will one day fly the nest to build a life of their own. Children and teenagers need their parents to be reliable, trustworthy and to provide a secure and stable platform from which they can step forward in their life and step back to when they need help or support.

The teenage years are a wonderful learning opportunity for the child and the parent. Both have to search deep inside to find their own resourcefulness and resilience to negotiate a path through challenging times. If parents try to be the perfect captain they fail to recognise that the sea of life is more powerful than any one individual. If however they practice mindfulness and work on their own wellness foundation they can weather the storms and be an ally to the teenager on their journey into adulthood.

It is an immense responsibility being a parent because children will look to you for guidance and support and they want you to honour their uniqueness as a person. As parents we make lots of mistakes and do not always recognise when we are failing to honour, respect or accept the child just as they are. It is human to err and if we recognise our mistakes and learn from each one it will help us to grow mentally and spiritually in our role as parents as well as human beings. There is no prize for parenting except the joy of seeing your child happy and living a fulfilled life. You cannot walk their life path but you can let them know you love them unconditionally no matter what storms you face.

Digging out the Roots

As people get older they tend to reflect on their life experiences including those associated with family. For many, the mid stage of their life appears to be a time when they feel ready to clear some of the emotional baggage from their past.

Perhaps a family bereavement, or children leaving home, or maybe the birth of a grandchild, has triggered old memories which they are now ready to process.

Alternatively, perhaps as you get older, you start to reflect on the meaning and purpose of life. As you do so, the need to clear some of the family related issues that you have silently carried for years, may emerge.

Irrespective of what the trigger is for such reflection and emotional clearing, it is an opportunity to let go of the past so that you can be spiritually and mentally free to enjoy the next stage of your life journey. I believe we are given only the experiences that we can handle and issues come up for clearing only when the person is ready to deal with them.

There is a societal expectation that family members will be loyal to each other, so when a family member shares with an 'outsider' about their negative experience, this can cause tension or perhaps a rift within the family. This is often the reason why family members do not open up to others about their difficult experiences.

Often however, when people do speak out about their past family experiences it is as though a dam has burst and the painful memories that have been held back for years come gushing out. Once these memories begin to flow, the healing process begins.

This is a form of spiritual awakening and presents an opportunity to uproot the cause of your pain, state your truth about how it affected you and then, consign it to the compost heap so that it can be transmuted into positive healing energy. A problem exists if you fail to clear, or continue to suppress your emotional wounds. By ignoring the roots of your pain you are denying your inner truth, and this will lead to dis-ease of the mind, body and spirit. Until the roots of pain are dug out and cleared, you will not blossom in wellness.

The emotional wounds of the past do not heal overnight but if they are carefully cleansed and then dressed with love, gentleness and forgiveness, healing can take place. For healing to occur you must learn to forgive those who have wounded you and if necessary detach from them until you are ready to reconcile. Forgiveness can be hard to offer because it is only necessary when we have been emotionally wounded by someone we care for or whom we believed cared for us. It is unusual to be hurt emotionally by someone you have no personal relationship with. Families have both a physical and emotional connection so it is especially painful when families hurt each other. The pain can go beyond the physical and your spirit may be deeply affected. I do not believe that the inner spirit can be broken but rather, that it fights for your survival during difficult times. Sadly however many people who have experienced deep emotional pain believe that their spirit has died and they become trapped in their pain. If they reach into the well of resilience inside themselves, they will see that they have the ability to move on from the wounds of the past, and to live a vibrant, loving and happy life.

Millions of people worldwide have lived through dreadful experiences including but not limited to, famine, disease, neglect, abuse, violence, torture, separation, abandonment, racism, poverty or forced migration. Yet many have moved on from these experiences with forgiveness and love in their hearts, instead of hatred or anger. Irrespective of whether their hurt or pain was caused by family members or strangers, they have been able to heal their lives and move forward in freedom and with inner peace.

They have done so because they choose to draw their spiritual and emotional energy from the fountain of love, forgiveness and reconciliation, and not from the painful well of the past. They are harvesters of healing love, and are positively energizing the wellness foundation of our planet.

For those who have been hurt by members of their family it is important that they confront their anger and pain and seek to heal it through forgiveness, compassion and love. This is something many will struggle with but in the interest of personal health and wellness it may be a life saving action. Sadly not everyone who has experienced hurt in the past is aware that they carry within themselves the power to heal their life. Instead they surrender to the darkness of anger, resentment or hate. Their spirit light fades and they seek to avoid or perhaps escape their life because they do not believe that they deserve, or will ever experience happiness and peace of mind.

Your spirit is not tangible matter and can recover from the deepest wounds and the darkest pain. This is because within you there is an infinite fountain of healing energy that seeks restoration of physical, spiritual and emotional harmony. If you draw your energy from this fountain, your spirit will be revived and your capacity for forgiveness, love, and wellness will expand.

Unless you give expression to your painful life experiences, the painful weeds will push their roots deeper into your heart, and will inhibit the expansion of wellness and serenity. If you cannot tell those who hurt you how you feel, then consider writing them a pain letter. Document how their behaviour wounded you, and describe in detail, its impact on your life. Let the words flow freely onto the page, and do not give into the temptation to edit the letter. This is your truth, your pain, and your story. It may take a number of letter writing sessions to clear all the pain and anger, so keep writing until you have expressed it all.

When there is nothing left to say, put the letter in an envelope and address it to those who have hurt you. You can choose to send the letter or, if you want to be emotionally and spiritually free, you can burn the letter and watch the pain of your past go up in flames. As the flames engulf the pages of pain in front of your eyes, take a deep breath and on the out breath release all of the pain, hurt and anger associated with your past experiences. Do this a number of time until the flame has disappeared and your body feels relaxed and at peace. Take a deep cleansing breath and give thanks for the freedom to have been able to dig out the stubborn roots of pain and to express your truth.

Some people may prefer to write a journal but you will need to consider what you are going to do with it when it is completed. If you put it in a drawer or somewhere out of sight you may feel that you have finished your healing work but that will not be the case. As long as the journal is there for you to read again, it will act as a reminder of the pain you have experienced and you will hold onto it despite your intent to let it go. Its roots will go deeper and continue to infect you spiritually and mentally.

Imagine a wound that has become infected. If you clean it and put on a dressing the healing process begins and you start to feel better. If you leave the same dressing on the wound it will fester and the infection will remain. To promote full healing, you must first cleanse the wound, dress it, and then change the dressing until such time as the infection is gone, the wound has healed and new skin has replaced what was once damaged and painful flesh. It is the same with your emotional wounds. You have to rid your emotional body of the infection that is caused by anger or resentment; otherwise it will imprison you and prevent you from finding peace and feeling love.

When you have finished your pain letters or journals and there is no more to be written or incinerated, it is time to start your letter or journal of gratitude. Start writing about the good things in your life and every day find at least one thing for which to be grateful. Perhaps someday you may express gratitude to those who hurt you, because this experience has helped you to recognise that you have within you the power to heal your life.

Healing and forgiveness is a gradual process and can be like ploughing a furrow so that a wellness crop can be planted. Your healing journey requires you to practice self care, develop self acceptance, be open to recognising love in others and accept that you are not responsible for what others have done to you. As you heal you will come to realise that those who hurt you were also hurting and while their behaviour was not acceptable, they may not have known any other way to act.

Past pain and anger has no place in your present or future life so dig it out, incinerate it and stop carrying it with you. All those hurtful experiences are absolutely in your past and although the people who were responsible for them may still be in your life you do not have to continue living your life defined by your past. By digging out the stubborn roots of pain you clear the way in your life for new experiences. When the poisonous roots of anger or resentment have been removed the ground becomes fertile and ready to be planted. Now you can look forward to an abundant harvest of wellness, wisdom and happiness

Sowing and Growing Wellness

As you work on healing your life, your relationship with your family will change and you will be able to detach from any hurt they may have contributed to. Some families are fantastic at supporting each other to heal their life, but others struggle to offer such support. As they see you change, some family members may view your changed behaviour or attitude as a rejection of them and they may be upset by this. Your family are not on the same personal life journey as you and unless you have shared with them about your decision to heal your life they may feel uncomfortable with this new you. After all you have behaved in a certain way for years and now suddenly you are changing the rules. Even though you are ready to soar like a butterfly or blossom like a flower your family may not be ready for any change to the status quo of their existence.

If a family is in conflict but someone within the family has an enduring illness or physical or mental health condition, the family may need the person to remain unwell so that the spotlight remains on them, thus detracting from other problems within the family. They may put their energies into focussing on the "sick" person rather than tending to the weeds in their own garden. Some may blame the pressure of living with or having to worry about a family member who is sick as the reason for their own problems. It is not uncommon to hear statements such as "If I did not have to worry about (the family member who is sick) I would not be so stressed" or "I would have a better social life" or "I could take on more responsibility at work" or similar declarations. Aspects of these may be true but the key to your wellness foundation is to take personal responsibility for your own wellness and healing and to garner support from those who will not undermine your efforts. In doing so you may have to respectfully detach from those who appear not to have your best interests at heart at this point in time.

A powerful antidote to family conflict is gratitude for the role each person plays within the family. When families focus on gratitude instead of conflict, positive relationships can develop and emotional wounds can be healed. The simple rules or guidelines you were taught as a child can help heal families and promote peace and harmony. These include saying please and thank you, asking permission, always tell the truth, owning up to your mistakes, apologising and making amends when you have done something wrong, showing respect toward others, avoiding being critical, sharing the workload, working as a team, taking turns, avoiding greed, generosity of spirit and saying your prayers. If families begin to apply these guidelines in daily life a lot of difficulties can be resolved, harmony can be achieved and wellness will blossom.

Each season brings new life to the garden. Seeds and bulbs are planted and shrubs and flowers grow and bloom. If not carefully tended the garden will become overgrown with weeds and the beautiful flowers and shrubs will wither and some will die. With careful cultivating, regular weeding and tender loving care, the garden will come alive with stunning colours and magical scents. The same is true with family. If we see family as a garden we will accept that there will always be weeds trying to disrupt peace and harmony. It is the personal responsibility of each family member to cultivate their own wellness patch and let it bloom. Once your wellness patch is in full bloom it may highlight the weeds in another part of the family garden, but it is not your job to fix this. Concentrate instead on minding what matters in the garden of your life. Invite others to spend time in your part of the family garden. By this I mean letting go of the past and extending the hand of friendship and love to your family so that the entire garden gets an opportunity to come alive and each flower within it can blossom.

Your job is not to change your family or convince them that your way is best. Your job is to work on your own wellness foundation and demonstrate respect for others who choose a different life path or garden design to you. Your life story can have a happy ever after if you let go of the pain of the past, embrace the gift of your life and express gratitude for your family. You cannot change your family but you can change your attitude toward them by remembering that they too are on a personal life journey and are doing the best they can. Wellness is like the unfolding petals of a lotus flower and as each one blossoms so too does wellness within the family.

PART THREE
The Inner Commentator

Your Personal Radio Station

Our brains are hardwired to process information which is translated into thoughts that in turn, influence our behaviour and attitude towards ourselves and others. The messages you receive from your family, friends, acquaintances, employers, colleagues, your community, from books and through the print and online media will have either a positive or negative impact on your thought process. If the messages you receive are predominately positive you will grown in confidence and you will go on to positively influence others you meet on your life journey. If on the other hand the messages you receive are primarily negative you may doubt your ability to be successful and your self esteem will be impaired. You may unconsciously create an inner dialogue that continuously reinforces these negative messages to the point where you accept them as being true.

Imagine that your mind is a radio station and the voice you hear is that of your inner commentator. Is the inner commentator applauding your unique gifts, abilities and the positives in your life or are they criticising your decisions, your feelings, your looks, your skills, your interests, your physical appearance, the sound of your voice and your ability to achieve your life goals? Does the inner commentator question your life choices and cause you to doubt yourself?

Most people at some stage have listened to live sports commentary on television or radio. The commentator plays a vital role in bringing the sporting action alive for the listener. Many of you will have a favourite sports commentator whom you tune in to regularly. Imagine if the sports commentator criticised every aspect of the game and the performance of every player from the start to the end of the game. Regardless of what team won the listener would probably switch off after the game feeling deflated. Chances are they would change channels for the next game. Imagine now if the same commentator was providing live coverage for every sports event that season and only one channel had the licence to broadcast. In this case the listener has limited options, either they put up with the negative commentary or they switch off for the entire season.

While this applies to commercial radio what about your own internal radio station. What is your inner commentator saying to you about you? Does your inner commentator build you up as a person or tear your down? Do they criticise everything you do or dismiss your achievements? Do they programme you to adopt a pessimistic outlook on life and pressure you to judge yourself harshly? Do they lobby you to make unfounded assumptions about yourself and other people? Or, is your inner commentator your advocate who encourages you to achieve your true potential in life, applauds your success, builds your self confidence and promotes wellness of your mind, body and spirit?

A negative dialogue from your inner commentator can lead to false beliefs which in turn lead to self defeating or self destructive behaviour. It is important to consider if your current beliefs and assumptions are true and how are these affecting your behaviour, attitude and ultimately your life satisfaction. If our predominant thoughts are negative and we identify with them they can become our inner beliefs. Thoughts are not real, they are just thoughts and if you continue to identify with negative thoughts you surrender your personal power and move away from wellness toward dis-ease of mind, body and spirit. It is important therefore to recognise that your thoughts only have the power that you give to them.

Likewise assumptions have no foundation unless you internalise them and turn them into beliefs. Becoming aware of the assumptions you make on a daily basis is essential when you are building your wellness foundation. Tune into the assumptions you make about yourself, other people or events in your life and consider what these assumptions are based on. In creating your wellness foundation it is important that you move toward not making assumptions about anyone or anything. This may require an ongoing effort but is extremely important if you wish to live a fulfilled and happy life.

Dr Michael Arloski PhD in his book *Wellness Coaching for Lasting Lifestyle Change* (2007) refers to the negative inner voice as the voice of the inner gremlin or inner critic. Irrespective of what you call your negative inner voice if you continue to give it permission to speak it will control your thinking, criticise your decisions and actions, condemn the way you look, berate your social skills and act like you personal inbuilt assailant. The negative inner commentator thrives on inner conflict and loves to hear you doubting yourself. It is driven by the desire to sabotage your efforts at finding inner peace and achieving personal life satisfaction. If you continue to give it air play it will prevent you from embracing wellness and will act as a permanent obstacle to your peace of mind.

Licence to Broadcast

Earlier I asked you to consider what vision you would have for a child as they embark on their life journey and how you could support them to fulfil this vision. Some of you will have identified that you would like the child to be confident, happy, have a positive self image and achieve their full potential. To support the child to realise this vision the adults in the child's life need be aware of the language or words they use when communicating with the child. If adults are respectful in how they communicate this will help the child to grow in self esteem.

Words, just like our thoughts can be powerful and can either build self esteem or undermine a persons' self worth. The words used to communicate with another person may have a harmful impact if they are negative and are spoken at a time when the person is emotionally vulnerable. We do not know when an individual is vulnerable to attacks on their self esteem so we should be mindful of the language we use in our interactions with others. If a child or adult is emotionally vulnerable and are subject to regular condemnation, criticism or other negative messages from significant people in their life, their self-image can become eroded. They may begin to believe they are worthless and may carry this belief throughout their life. Negative beliefs about oneself provide ammunition for the inner commentator and the script for negative self talk begins to be written.

Messages communicated to children, either positive or negative, can have a long term impact on their self esteem. Many people I have spoken to can recall a particular message communicated to them in childhood by an adult or older child that became life defining for them. Some of these messages were positive and gave the child the confidence to pursue their life goals and give expression to their dreams and ambitions. Others however were negative and had a lasting effect on the person's confidence throughout their childhood, adolescence and on into adulthood. Critical comments recalled by some include, "you are good for nothing", "you are stupid", "you are always messing up", "you are such a disappointment to me", "I am ashamed of you" or "you will never amount to anything." Such messages have the potential to have a profoundly adverse effect on a persons' self worth.

When a persons' self worth is eroded they do not value their own achievements or capabilities, often have low levels of life satisfaction and may fail to recognise the greatness that they are capable of. They can feel under constant pressure to project an outward image of being in control despite being in emotional pain. Others wear a mask to avoid revealing their real self to others because they fear being negatively judged by others. Many need support to heal the emotional wounds of the past, but may be too afraid or, too ashamed to ask for help. Imagine spending your life filled with self loathing and never experiencing inner happiness. Imagine having to wear a mask that says everything is fine in your life when in fact the opposite is true. Imagine the mental, physical and spiritual pain the person experiences every day and how this impacts on their health and wellness. Imagine that no matter what you achieved you never believed it was enough and you never experienced contentment or inner peace.

Undoubtedly there are millions of people who have heard negative messages during their lives but did not absorb them. This is most likely because they were not emotionally vulnerable at the time these messages were conveyed and consequently their lives have not been defined by such messages. Sadly though, many others live their lives in accordance with the negative messages they heard and never feel happy or fulfilled.

Others may have developed an addiction which by its nature will continuously reinforce their negative self image and serve to maintain their low self esteem. Common experiences of those living with an addiction include a lack of self love, personal shame, a deeply ingrained sense of worthlessness and a difficulty in establishing trusting relationships. Some of the people I have met who have experienced addiction spoke about the critical broadcasts from their inner commentator. These serve to reinforce their belief that they were worthless and cause them to feel deeply ashamed of whom they believe themselves to be. They seek to escape this mental torment through food, alcohol, gambling or other forms of addiction. Addiction however is not a form of escape but rather a state of imprisonment. In some way those who experience addiction are punishing themselves because they believe themselves to be worthless. The dis-ease that arises from addiction is quite powerful. It strips away the person's self esteem and erodes their wellness foundation. Social connection and support is a core building block for wellness, but for some people this building block can often seem beyond their reach.

Even when a persons' emotional wellness has been undermined their inner spirit will fight for survival and if they reach out for support their wellness journey can began. If they connect with others in their time of need they can re-build their lives, begin to recognise their value as a human being, find inner peace, and experience personal freedom and wellness. It is never too late to change the script of the inner commentator and as you do you will begin to develop self worth and reclaim your personal power.

Towards a New Script

Think for a minute about building a house. Would a wise person build it on wet land or on dry ground? For a house to last a lifetime it needs a solid and stable foundation. The same is true for wellness. If however, you allow the negative inner commentator to be the architect of your life choices then your wellness foundation will be unstable. Furthermore you may never find inner peace or fulfil your life ambitions or dreams. You have the ability to change the script of your inner commentator but first you must reclaim your personal power and direct that power toward championing wellness and self love.

Perhaps you once were a vulnerable child and someone in your life without conscious intent to harm passed a critical comment toward you or about you. Unconsciously you may have developed a belief that what they said was true and perhaps you began to you live your life accordingly. You cannot have personal freedom until you know your own truth. By this I mean the inner truth of who you really are and not some false belief based on what others have said to you, or about you. Living according to a false truth prevents you from revealing the inner you and recognising that you are an amazing person with a divine life purpose. It is time to let your inner light radiate outwards by finding within yourself the absolute truth of who you are. You are a divine child of the universe, and your worth is beyond measure. With courage and effort you can challenge your negative beliefs, silence the negative voice of the inner commentator and replace it with positive self talk.

You get to choose from this point forward the language you use when you talk to yourself, and to others. For the sake of your physical, mental and spiritual wellness make sure the language you use is positive and truthful. No more lies to yourself about yourself, no more masking your inner truth and no more self criticism. You are good enough, you can achieve more than you ever imagined, you deserve to love and be loved, you deserve respect, you deserve a healthy mind and body, you deserve to feel good about yourself, you are capable and competent, you are uniquely special, and you are beautiful. In time you will develop the confidence to say these things to yourself. But for now, start to gently change the script of the inner commentator, to one that is uplifting, instead of one that drags you down.

Will your life ever be perfect? The answer to this question depends on how you define perfect. If you start living according to your inner truth which includes your choices, your moral beliefs, your wellness vision and your core values, then I believe your life will be as perfect as it is destined to be. It may not be easy at times but you will restore balance in your life and on this you will build your personal wellness foundation. If you try to live according to others people's standards, beliefs and values and these are not aligned to your own, there will be an imbalance in your life and you will struggle to achieve inner peace. As you systematically change your inner dialogue, you will start to enjoy your life journey, and look forward to the next stage of the adventure.

It is unlikely that the negative inner commentator will disappear completely. However, when you develop conscious awareness of its existence, and reclaim your personal power, the voice of truth will take over the broadcast. Adopting positive self talk requires effort and determination, but you will feel the benefits as your confidence and self worth grows. Some people are capable of changing the script of the inner commentator, and sowing the seeds for wellness, with the support of family or friends. Others however, may need a more formal support structure to get started and to stay on track. There is no shame in wanting to be happy so ask for help and then go forth and harvest your inner truth and blossom in wellness and wisdom.

PART FOUR
The Fountain of Truth- Cornerstones of Wellness

Beyond the Mask

Relationships are a central element of human existence and strongly influence our wellness foundation. Because this is your personal life journey, your primary relationship is with yourself. Secondary to this are the relationships you form with other people including family, friends, and acquaintances.

You will have a positive relationship with some people, have a neutral relationship with others, and perhaps have a challenging relationship with some of those you meet along the way. Each relationship is important for your personal growth, and you do not know when you first meet someone, what life lessons they have to offer you.

Some people carry a lot of anger or resentment and their behaviour toward you or others may appear aggressive, rude or even abusive. Others may be overtly critical or may lie, bully or manipulate others in order to exert control. The person who displays this type of behaviour is in conflict with their inner self, and unless they resolve this they will be at war with the world. This is their war, not yours so be careful not to get caught up in their conflict.

Those who carry the burden of anger, often lack inner peace, and find it difficult to offer a genuine compliment or a word of praise to others. Often they are unwilling to accept responsibility for their personal situation, or to make an effort to improve it. They may blame the government, their family, a partner, the education system, their employer, the economy, or perhaps God, for their perceived problems.

Often they are convinced that they are right and everyone else is wrong. This world view places them in a consistently defensive position as they journey through life. Often they have little insight as to how their negative behaviour affects other people. Without such insight they have difficulty sustaining loving relationships, and miss out on the mental and spiritual wellness that comes from connecting in a meaningful way, with other people.

Behind their mask of hostility or aggression they may lack self confidence and may actually feel powerless. Many seek to reclaim power by trying to control those around them. They do not realise that personal power is owned when you stop trying to be in control and surrender instead to love, forgiveness, peace and harmony. Those who carry a burden of anger and resentment have unknowingly placed obstacles on their own path to wellness and inner peace. They are like the delicate rose that has become entangled in the briars of life and their inner beauty is not shining through.

If you have experienced the wrath of such people you are unlikely to have much sympathy for them. Remember however, that at some point along their life journey, they tuned out of the voice of truth, and tuned into the voice of negativity, fear and anger. Their personal life experiences, will have influenced their behaviour and attitude. If they have had painful experiences in the past, this may have contributed to the burden of negative emotions they are carrying. These people need empathy and support to reignite the inner light that reflects who they really are. Only when they allow their inner light to shine through can it dispel the dark shadow that hangs over them.

Some may never change their behaviour or attitude, and might remain angry with the world. This is their choice, so let them be, and focus instead on building your own wellness foundation. Be grateful for the life lessons albeit painful that they have taught you. Detach from them without judgement, wish them well and move forward on your own path to wellness.

From a Place of Love

Universal wellness is a direct reflection of the level of wellness experienced by each individual living on planet earth. Wellness and positive energy are intertwined and when you are well, you emit a glowing energy which reflects your life force. Your life force energy affects those you come into contact with and the stronger your wellness foundation the more powerful your life force energy will be. When your life force energy is powered by love this will energise those you meet. Love is a powerful force and universal wellness can be strengthened through one small act of love at a time. When we operate from a place of love we can move emotional mountains and build bridges of harmony among families, communities and across nations. Universal wellness is possible if each person commits to nurturing their own wellness foundation and sharing the gift of love with those they meet.

Never underestimate your contribution toward universal wellness. Compare the impact that love and forgiveness has on the wellness of the global population versus the effects of anger and hatred. As humans we have capacity for great acts of love but also capacity for acts that do great harm. It is tragic to see how much pain human beings inflict on each other as is evident in the many wars occurring in our precious world today. Every act of war or terrorism, irrespective of where or why it occurs, is a barrier to the wellness of all humanity. Whenever one person on planet earth is hurt by others, their life force is weakened, and this weakens the life force of the planet.

War and human conflict is often driven by fear based anger, hatred, feelings of oppression, unresolved guilt and emotional wounds from past experiences. So many children, parents, brothers, sisters, aunts, uncles, cousins and grandparents die every day because mankind has not figured out a peaceful and loving way to overcome fear, anger, guilt, hatred and oppression.

If you feel oppressed by a person's behaviour you may react in anger. An angry response will not resolve the issue, and is likely to make matters worse. Even though you might justify your reaction, you often end up hurting yourself more than the person on the receiving end of your anger. If your mind, body and spirit are filled with anger and hate this poison will infiltrate every cell of your body, your life force energy will weaken and you will move away from wellness toward dis-ease and illness. You may believe that by getting even with, or by punishing someone, for harm they have caused, that you will feel better about the situation. This will not be the case, because your anger will continue to poison your body and mind, until such time as you let it go.

You can learn to articulate your truth directly and respectfully without demeaning another person. By doing this you will have completed a small but significant act of truth that will positively influence the universal life force and your own wellness foundation. If for just one day every human being on our planet earth expressed their truth without intent to hurt others, the positive effect on the earths' energy would be powerful and wellness and harmony among all living things would begin to be restored.

This is our world, these are our people and we collectively determine the level of individual, community and universal wellness that exists at any given time. Your starting point is conducting one small act of love toward yourself and then moving on to those whom you are in relationship with, including your family and community.

Freedom through Gratitude

Your mindset determines your life choices and when it is underpinned by gratitude you are free to make healthy life choices. A positive outlook and gratefulness for the simple things in life will carry you through difficult life events. Those who freely express gratitude have chosen a life path lined with appreciation and forgiveness. They have let go of the emotional baggage they have been carrying, and in doing so have reclaimed their personal freedom.

Many people who experience a serious or life limiting illness go on to adopt a positive and gratitude filled attitude toward life. They have the W (Wellness) factor and come to accept their illness with grace and humility and draw strength from their spiritual beliefs. They demonstrate how to live well until they die. This mindset helps them prioritise the things that are most important in their life. This may include spending quality time with family and friends, contributing to their community, adopting a healthier lifestyle or focusing on their spiritual development. They place their medical or surgical treatment in the hands of doctors but take personal responsibility for their emotional or spiritual healing. They trust their doctors, their God and their body to do what is necessary for their physical, mental or spiritual wellness and recovery. They believe in their ability to face whatever the outcome is and express gratitude for the life they have been granted. They believe that their illness has given them the opportunity to take stock of their lives and to start living mindfully and in accordance with their inner truth. Even though they may have a life limiting condition they blossom in wellness and share this with those they meet along the way.

When serious illness strikes, not everyone will be able to view this as an opportunity to reflect on the good they have experienced in their life. Many live their lives in hope but with a limited sense of gratitude. Hope is wonderful thing to have but gratitude is equally important in shaping our lives. Hope is an expression of a desire whereas gratitude is an expression of an achievement. Rather than saying "I hope I do not die" one might instead say "I am grateful to be alive today and there is so much I can still do before I die."Many people spend their lives hoping they will not get sick or that they will not lose their job or, that a relationship will work out or, that they will find the money to pay that overdue bill or, that a sick family member will recover. Yes, we must have hope and be optimistic because without hope we may feel like giving up. However it is important to recognise that we are not helpless in these situations. If we recognise and express gratitude for what we can do when faced with adverse life events we will reclaim our personal power and not leave it all to hope or chance.

Many of those who have had painful life experiences, find it difficult to feel, or to express gratitude. However, by acknowledging one thing each day that you are grateful for, you will maintain a focus on the positive aspects of your life. This can be particularly helpful when you are struggling with a personal challenge. Without gratitude you are likely to feel resentment when life gets tough. Resentment once it takes hold leaves little room for serenity. Resentment is a heavy burden to carry and could easily be lightened if you begin to look for things to be thankful for in your life.

We all know people who exude positive energy and others whose energy seems to drain us. I like being around energy lifters rather than the energy drainers. People who regularly express gratitude and offer forgiveness are energy lifters and have a positive effect on those around them. Strive to be an energy lifter and identify at least one thing each day to be grateful for, regardless of how small or insignificant it may seem. In doing so you begin to dis-empower resentment and move toward wellness and greater life satisfaction.

Yes, life can be very tough, and at times it can feel cruel. However there are only two certainties in life, firstly that we will live and secondly that we will die. One day your life journey will end and when it does there is no going back to change the past. Each day offers us a chance to start over, so just for today choose gratitude, choose forgiveness and choose wellness. There is always something to be grateful for even when you are struggling and in pain, so dig deep and find it, express it and hold onto it.

Farewell Judge and Jury

Each of us is a unique spiritual being on a personal journey of discovery through which we can develop conscious awareness and fulfil our life purpose. On this journey we get to unlock the fountain of truth and wisdom inside ourselves and this allows us to blossom in physical, mental and spiritual wellness.

Your life journey will present you with a series of tough but essential lessons along the way. At times these lessons will be difficult. However, if you are open to learning, you will gradually discover your inner truth, and you will come to know who you really are, at the very core of your being. It is not always easy to acknowledge and accept ourselves and at times we may be tempted to ignore the aspects of ourselves that we are uncomfortable with or which we do not like. However to be spiritually well we must come to accept ourselves just as we are. Criticism and harsh judgement of oneself or others is an obstacle to spiritual wellness. Yet judging ourselves or others often by unrealistic and unattainable standards is a common human trait. A judgemental attitude can result in us becoming locked into a cycle of criticism leaving little room for appreciation and praise.

Often times we find it difficult to acknowledge or applaud the achievements of others and this may also be true of ourselves. When you are critical of yourself or others, your life force energy becomes dense, and others will not want to be around you. Equally if a person near you is overtly critical, their energy will be dense, and you will feel the need to withdraw from their company. This is a protection strategy adopted by the spirit because it recognises the lower energy of another person as something that will undermine your wellness foundation. Think about the people you come into contact with in your everyday life. How many of these give off a negative vibe or leave you eager to escape their company? We are surrounded by negative energy every day, primarily because many people have spiritual dis-ease instead of spiritual wellness.

Children from an early age become programmed to judge, condemn and criticise themselves and others. If you live with criticism you are likely to become critical, if you live with harsh judgement you are likely to judge yourself and others harshly, and if you live with condemnation you are likely to condemn yourself or others. On the other hand if you live with praise you learn to accept and give praise, and if you are shown respect then you learn to respect yourself and others. Look at a group of children and spot the ones who have a positive life force that exudes love, shows respect for other, and basks in happiness and contentment. These are the ones with whom other children want to play and they are like rays of sunshine. We can all find our inner ray of light and get rid of the dark shadow of spiritual dis-ease we sometimes carry around. This takes work and requires a mindset shift from being critical and judgmental, to being accepting of, and respectful toward others.

There would be a phenomenal shift in the earth's energy if every individual on this planet stopped judging others and choose instead to express appreciation and gratitude, adopted a positive outlook on their life, demonstrated respect towards themselves and others and committed to seeing something good in everyone who crossed their path.

Getting to the Truth of the Matter

Now is the right time to reclaim your personal power and take responsibility for your life choices. There is nothing helpful to be gained from blaming others for your past pain or current situation. Yes, others may have contributed to your pain by their words or actions, and perhaps you have been deeply wounded by them. However, by holding onto anger or resentment you will continue to experience emotional pain and this will block your path to wellness.

There are people in all of our lives whom by their behaviour or words have given us genuine cause to feel anger or resentment.

Regardless of whether it was intentional or not you must accept that you are not responsible for their behaviour or words, nor can you change them. You are solely responsible for how you behave and what you say. If you choose anger you have to understand that this anger will hurt you more than the person it is directed toward. Anger and resentment will take you to a dark place where you are driven to say or do things in an attempt to get even with, or punish others. Letting go of anger, finding forgiveness and where possible reconciling with those who have offended or hurt you is an antidote to emotional and spiritual pain.

If you choose to act from a place of love you can do no harm. Love is the most powerful source of fuel for your life force energy and without love this world would be a darker place. Just as I have suggested that you express gratitude for one thing every day I would also suggest that you express love toward at least one person each day through word or deed. Through daily acts of love you will begin to experience inner peace and serenity, which is what spiritual wellness is ultimately about. You deserve peace and harmony in your life but until you clear your body, mind and spirit of anger and resentment you will not achieve this.

Every person on this earth has within them the power to fulfil their spiritual potential and to live a happy, meaningful and well balanced life. For many people this requires a release of intolerance, resentment, judgement, false assumptions and a letting go of the need to be in control. It requires an acknowledgement that you have within you a higher energy that reflects your capacity for great acts of goodness but you also carry a lower energy which, if in control draws you away from wellness. This lower energy is powered by negative thoughts and behaviours including dishonesty, jealousy, criticism, disrespect, gossip and intolerance of others.

Enhancing your spiritual wellness requires you to hold up a mirror to this part of yourself and acknowledge that it exists. Once you recognise this truth you can begin to nurture your higher self through respect, compassion, forgiveness, praise and self acceptance. If anger, hurt, resentment or hate are current obstacles on your path to spiritual wellness now is the time to start removing them. As you draw from the fountain of truth inside yourself your wellness foundation will be strengthened and you will reap the rewards of harmony, love and serenity in your life.

PART FIVE
Turning Obstacles into Building Blocks

Wellness beyond Grief

Our physical, mental and spiritual wellness is influenced by many factors including past experiences, stress, relationships, social and community connections, personal motivation, finance, current physical and mental health, access to resources and support, self efficacy, your attitude toward your personal health, grief and loss and your readiness to make changes in your life. This is not an exhaustive list, but these along with many other influencing factors, will hold different levels of importance at various stages of your life. Some factors such as death, or the loss or deterioration of physical or mental health cannot be accurately predicted in terms of when they will occur.

Grief is equated with loss and may be linked to the death of a family member, a friend, a colleague, the loss of an important personal relationship, loss of health, financial loss, loss of security in terms of your home or your job, children leaving home, or for others, the loss of a much loved pet.

There are many losses that people experience throughout their life but not all losses result in grief therefore it is important to make this distinction. The onset of a serious illness, or the death of a loved one, may shake the very core of your wellness foundation. At such times you may feel utterly disconnected, from any sense of life satisfaction or inner peace. Indeed you may temporarily move away from wellness and toward dis-ease of mind, body and spirit as you come to terms with a life altering event. Grief is a personal journey and each individual will experience it at varying levels of intensity and move through the grieving process at different rates. It is possible that in the early stages of grief you may not feel motivated to engage in positive lifestyle practices and survival, not wellness may be your primary focus.

When someone close to you dies or acquires a serious illness or disability there is a deep sense of loss and you have to allow yourself time to grieve this loss. If it is you who has acquired a disability or a serious illness then the sense of loss is likely to be more profound. Life as you have known it has changed fundamentally and you may feel powerless, and afraid that you will never get through this difficult time. Parents whose children are born with or develop a life limiting condition grieve twice. Firstly they grieve the loss of the anticipated healthy baby and then when their child dies they grieve the loss of the child who has graced their lives albeit for a short time.

Many people who are diagnosed with a serious or life threatening health condition do go on to make significant life changes once they have accepted their diagnosis. They learn that they can thrive not just survive in the face of adversity. Many embrace a healthier lifestyle and become more mindful in how they live from that point onwards. Even though they have experienced the loss of full health or a terminal diagnosis, they recognise this as an opportunity to reclaim other aspects of their health and wellness as they embark on the remainder of their life journey. So even though grief arising from a significant loss is painful it can present an opportunity to evaluate your life and adopt a new perspective. It may be painful, exhausting and at times frustrating, but you have within you, the resilience to cope with whatever you face on this uncharted life journey.

Life is filled with expectations, hopes and dreams and when a loved one dies or becomes ill it can feel like these all disappear in an instant. Some people find it difficult to see a future beyond their loss. When this occurs the wellness foundation of the person is eroded and they feel physically, emotionally and spiritually empty. Irrespective of how dark life seems, your wellness foundation is never beyond repair. Unfortunately however many find it difficult to reach out for help or are unable to speak about how they are feeling. The saddest thing is when someone chooses not to seek help or tries to hide their pain, and then one day it becomes too heavy a burden and they stop choosing life. They may find peace in leaving their pain behind but the world mourns the loss of one of its brightest lights.

This world needs all of us for it to be complete. Maybe right now you do not realise how much your very existence contributes to this world and the people in it. You are more than a number, more than a son or daughter, more than a parent, more than a brother or sister, an aunt or uncle, a grandparent, a cousin, a friend, a neighbour, a colleague, the boss, a priest, a coach, a minister, a healer, or whatever other title or role you hold. You are more than any title. You are a child of the universe with a life purpose which when fulfilled will allow you to blossom in wellness and wisdom and in doing so make this world a better place. If you choose not to be here then you do not fulfil that purpose and the world suffers the loss of your contribution.

If you are struggling with loss or grief and you are finding it difficult to cope, you can reach out to others who will walk with you, hold your hand and support you through your difficult times. Your life journey is paved with challenges but also beautifully lined with friendship and support. Do not resist reaching out to others for support because one day you will be in a position to reciprocate it for someone else. It is through this mutual support that we build our universal wellness foundation.

The lack of certainty in life, and perhaps a fear of the unknown is the reason why many people look to psychics or fortune tellers, to predict their future. If we all knew today what the future has in store for us we would spend our time anticipating the events to come but perhaps missing out on what we already have. There is nothing wrong with looking to the future but you cannot live there, you can only live in the present. While no-one knows for certain what the future holds one thing that is guaranteed is that each of us will die at some point. With this in mind we should embrace life, live well until we die and enjoy the journey moment by moment and day by day.

Who Put the Knot in Your Can?

When it comes to taking action to improve their health and wellness, many people craft excuses for why they cannot make a change. Excusitis should be labelled a chronic condition because it seems to flare up when we are about to embark on a lifestyle change or when we are implementing a change and struggling to maintain it. The excuses may vary but they usually start with *"I cannot"* and it seems like we have tied a knot in our self belief by adding *"not"* to the end of *"I can"*.

Commonly used excuses include; I cannot lose weight because I have a slow metabolism; I cannot stick to this diet because I am always hungry; I cannot exercise because I do not have time; I cannot quit smoking because I will put on weight; I cannot give up chocolate because I am addicted; I cannot start an exercise class because I have no one to mind the children; I cannot go for a walk today because it is too wet; I cannot ask for a raise because I know they will say no; I cannot say no to the extra work because I am on a temporary contract; I cannot take a lunch break because I have too much work to do; I cannot help out with the fundraiser because I hate asking people for money; I cannot have this conversation with my partner because I know they will get angry; I cannot attend church because I like to relax on a Sunday morning; I cannot stop playing computer games because I am trying to get to the next level; I cannot go to bed early because this is when my favourite TV programme is on or, I just cannot say no to others. Sound familiar?

When you say *"I can"* it means you have made a decision to take action based on a desired outcome. However if your default mindset is *"I cannot"*, then you have tied a knot in your belief, that you have the ability, or capacity, to take action. When children say that they cannot do something, for example riding a bicycle, they have an expectation of failure. Unless they are encouraged and taught to cycle, they will not master the skill and will internalize the belief that they cannot ride a bicycle. This lowers their personal expectations and self-confidence.

Perhaps along your life journey you were not supported, or encouraged, to master new skills, or to pursue your dreams. This may have eroded your self esteem and caused you to give up on your goals or ambitions. Certainly others do influence our thinking and attitudes, but we ourselves have the ultimate power to change our mindset, and make the shift from the *"I cannot"* to the *"I can"* frame of mind. It is time to untie the knot that is preventing you from achieving your full potential in life.

There may be valid reasons why you cannot commit to something but there may also be veiled excuses that are presented as reasons. If for example you are considering running a marathon next month and your inner commentator is telling you that you cannot do so because you have not started training, then this is a valid point worth listening to. You do not have to dismiss your goal but instead focus on making it more realistic and attainable. If on the other hand, you want to increase your physical activity, but your inner commentator is saying you are too old or some other excuses, then you need to recognise that a mindset shift is required. The key is to differentiate between a valid reason and an actual excuse. Sometimes we view things as obstacles because we are afraid to make a change. It is time to expose the excuses you make, stop feeding your fear of change, and get on with living a happy and fulfilled life.

As you embark on improving your health and wellness you will need to adopt the belief that you can do whatever you set your mind to. This self belief has the effect of dis-empowering fear. Remember, fear only has power, if you surrender to fear. Self belief sounds something like this, I can lose weight; I can incorporate regular physical activity into my life; I can feed my family a healthy diet on a limited budget; I can learn to cook; I can quit smoking; I am not too old to adopt a healthy lifestyle; I can be healthy and well and I can support my family to do the same.

I can, is all about personal choices and decisions. You get to choose every day which direction to go, and what changes you want to make to your life or lifestyle. If you really want to enjoy your life, choose health, choose wellness and choose happiness. Then start to dismantle the obstacles that impede your progress.

A Different Outlook

Obstacles to physical, mental or spiritual wellness may include physical or mental health disorders, illness or disability, grief and loss or other significant life events. Even though physical or mental illness or disability do creates certain challenges to our quality of life there are still many choices that can be made to improve your overall health and wellness. Recently I meet a mother and her adult daughter at a swimming pool. The young lady was a wheelchair user and as her mother helped her into the pool it was apparent that she loved being in the water. Her mother explained to me that her daughter has physical, sensory and intellectual impairments but loves going to the gym, swimming and getting out in the fresh air, particularly to the beach and the woods. Her mother viewed these experiences as being vital to her daughter's happiness and wellbeing, and so did not let her disabilities hold her back from enjoying life. We only have to look at the Paralympics and Special Olympic games to see that people with disabilities can overcome many barriers to achieve their personal goals and fulfil their life ambitions. Yet as a society we regularly create physical and social barriers for people with disabilities and or mental health difficulties.

Health is not just physical and it is not possible to examine physical health and wellness without giving consideration to your mental and spiritual health and wellness. If you are mentally and emotionally well you are more likely to give attention to your physical health and be motivated to adopt healthy food choices, take regular exercise, practice mindfulness and manage stress in your life. In other words you are more likely to take responsibility for your health.

If you are mentally or emotionally unwell then you may find it difficult to motivate yourself to look after your health or to achieve balance in your life. It is important therefore, when contemplating any lifestyle change, to consider the physical, psychological, emotional or spiritual challenges that may impact on your ability to sustain the change. This includes your outlook on life and your motivation to change.

Our outlook or mindset can be a stubborn obstacle to wellness and life satisfaction. Think for a moment about your attitude to your own health and wellness. Do you see yourself as being responsible for maintaining your health or is it outside of your control? Until we change our outlook and accept responsibility for our personal health and wellness we will always find excuses dressed up as obstacles as to why we cannot make life or lifestyle changes.

Eat Well to Feel Well

Because none of us know what our lifespan will be, it is important to live well until we die. This includes respecting your body, nourishing and hydrating it with healthy food and fluids, exercising it regularly, resting it when it is tired and allowing it time to heal when it is injured. The human body needs fuel so that it can function well in accordance with what it is designed to do. When the fuel it receives via food and drink is healthy then the body operates efficiently. If however you consume unhealthy processed food and drinks on an ongoing basis your body will underperform, your energy levels will be low, your sleep will be disrupted, your breathing and heart rate may be affected and the engines of your cells will not function at peak performance. You cannot expect excellent health if you treat your body with low quality fuel. If you bought a new car you would expect it to run smoothly without any engine problems. If you put the correct fuel into it and have it serviced regularly you could expect that it will continue to run efficiently. Over time as the car gets older you will have to give it extra care and replace some of its parts. Eventually you will have to trade it in for a replacement model.

Now what about your body? It is without doubt the most magnificent vehicle you will ever own with a potentially long lifespan. If properly cared for it will serve you well throughout your childhood, adolescence, adulthood and your older years until it is ready to retire. Some people however will get sick or acquire life limiting illnesses and die young despite having lived a healthy lifestyle. This is the nature of your personal life journey and we must recognise that some things are simply out of our control.

Obesity is fast becoming a global epidemic, is shortening the lifespan of millions of adults and children and is significantly increasing the cost of health care provision. If you do the grocery shopping in your home do you shop with a view to buying ingredients for a healthy diet or do you choose processed and convenience foods because they are cheaper and less time consuming to prepare? Convenience foods and drinks are called convenient for many reasons. They tend to require little effort to prepare and this conveniently results in less preparation and cooking time and also less washing up. Unfortunately they are not a convenient way to support nutritional health.

Advertising may lead you to believe that fruit juice contributes to one of your daily portions of fruit. In reality, it is more likely to offer unnecessary spoons of sugar to your body, which have no health benefits. Processed foods and drinks tend to be high in sugar or salt and low in vitamins and minerals required for healthy growth and development. When you consume highly processed foods on an ongoing basis, your digestive system does not function at its optimum and your liver, pancreas and kidneys work overtime to deal with the toxic overload from a high sugar, high salt and sometimes additive laced diet. Excess sugar is converted to, and stored as fat in the abdominal wall, around the organs, and some remains in your blood. This increases your risk of coronary heart disease, diabetes and stroke. Ultimately a highly processed diet is a recipe for physical ill health and will increase your risk of chronic disease in later life.

With affluence comes time pressures and in the last few decades we have witnessed a move away from growing our own fruit and vegetables and looking to nature for our primary source of food. Previous generations worked in unison with nature to feed their families. They grew their own grains, vegetables and potatoes, reared their own chickens, cows, pigs, goats and sheep and in doing so had a fresh supply of milk, eggs, meat, grains, poultry and vegetables to feed their family. Those living near rivers or the coast fished and had a diet that included high quality protein loaded with healthy fish oils. Life was tough and the work was hard but the alternative was starvation as there were few or no supermarkets, convenience stores or fast food outlets.

Over time with industrialisation people began to rely less directly on the land and sea for their food supply and the era of convenience and processed food began in earnest. Today many children grow up not knowing where the fruits and vegetables they see in supermarkets have originally come from. It seems that over time in western society we have sacrificed physical wellness for convenience, and now we are paying the health price. Thankfully there is a move back toward growing your own produce and farmers markets are an example of the success of this. If you live in a city or apartment block you can argue that you have no space to grow your own food. This is true if you want to grow a large supply of fruit or vegetables, but pots of herbs on your window sill are a starting point or investing in a community allotment is another option. If you cannot grow your own vegetables or fruit at least aim to buy produce that resembles what it looked like when it was growing in nature.

We know that an unhealthy diet is an obstacle to physical wellness but so too is limited finance. While many in our society are affluent there are many more trying to survive on a low income with a limited amount of money to spend on food. Some people who are experiencing food poverty may lack knowledge about nutrition and therefore buy processed food due to a lack of awareness of the alternatives. It is important that those experiencing food poverty are supported through dietary education including simple guides to healthy shopping and preparing healthy meals on a limited budget. Others may be knowledgeable about nutrition and healthy eating but buy cheaper processed foods simply because they have a limited income. Healthy food choices can still be made on a restricted budget but it takes some advance planning. You need to plan your weekly menu and then make your grocery shopping list based on this menu. Shops and supermarkets regularly have special offers on meat, fish, vegetables, fruit, grains or other ingredients that support a healthy diet. Become a smart shopper and look out for these special offers.

Your daily diet is the fuel source for your body so view it in a positive light, choose healthful foods and make water your beverage of choice as often as you can. Once you get into the habit of making healthy food choices you need never again go on a restrictive diet. Food is for enjoyment as well as being a fuel source. You and your body are a match literally made in heaven so love it and treat it well. Even when you experience ill health your body will seek recovery and repair so let it do its job and stop putting barriers in its way. Would you put mud in the engine of your car and expect it to run smoothly? Of course not, so why would you fill your fabulous body with junk food and sugary drinks and still expect it to work well for you? Learn to listen to your body because it knows exactly what it needs to serve you well. Give it the best chance for longevity and it will carry you carefully on your personal life journey. If your body is healthy on the inside your will feel great and look amazing and that, arguably is a wellness recipe worth trying.

Wellness in Motion

Regular exercise supports positive physical, mental and spiritual wellness. However advancements in technology including transport, television, computer games and social media, coupled with an increase in sedentary occupations, has contributed to adults and children becoming less physically active. I do not dispute the fact that in many countries children and adults are sufficiently physically active to support positive health. However from a universal health perspective we all need to exercise more often and for longer periods of time. Non participation in regular physical activity coupled with an increasingly high sugar and highly processed diet is contributing to the growing epidemic of obesity and other lifestyle diseases including cardiovascular disease, certain cancers and diabetes.

Our bodies are designed to be in motion from the day we are born. If you watch a baby you will notice that when they are awake they are either moving or making efforts to move. At every stage of a child's development they strive to move because this is what their body is designed to do. It goes against natures design to be inactive. The good news is that within each of us is a natural born exerciser, which may, over time have become latent. The challenge is to resurrect the exerciser within and re-ignite your motivation to move. Exercise and physical activity should be incorporated within your daily routine and not be viewed as an add-on. Regular exercise is a key component of the care package for your body, and when combined with a healthy diet will support your physical and mental health.

Regardless of what the initial driver to start exercising is, many people lose interest or motivation after a period of time and often revert to being a non exerciser. To avoid this pitfall it is important to have a clear vision of what you want to achieve from exercising, including, the value it will add to your quality of life. Your vision should describe what your body will look like and feel like when you are fit and healthy. For example you may envision that when you are fit your body will be strong and toned, you will have lost weight, you will have increased stamina and you will feel confident and look great. The fun part, believe it or not, is exercising to make this vision a reality. If you do not have a vision for what you want to achieve from regular exercise, chances are you will not place a high value on exercising and this will affect your motivation and commitment. Without personal motivation and a commitment to your vision you will find it difficult to sustain regular exercise. So start with a vision underpinned by the value it will bring to your life, support this with a commitment to exercise and then go ahead and take action through your preferred type of exercise or physical activity.

Consider for a moment how you feel when you sit in front of the television versus how you feel when you have just come back from a swim, run, cycle, game of football, tennis match, walk in the fresh air or whatever type of exercise you engage in. Your head will be clearer after exercising and you will feel more alive inside, whereas if you sit on the couch for long periods of time you will feel lethargic and your balance will also be affected.

Aside from supporting weight loss, improving muscle tone and strength and increasing your overall physical fitness, exercise is also a great stress buster. When you exercise, feel good hormones are released and these enhance your mental and emotional wellness. Many will argue that chocolate has a similar effect, but although it may taste delicious and it may temporarily lift your mood it will not lift sagging muscles, burn fat or improve your level of fitness. Neither does chocolate help clear the mind or support you to cope with the stress and challenges you are presented with in life.

It is said that a fit body supports a fit mind. A fit mind means you are clear in your thinking and decision making and your brain does not feel like it is fogged up. How many times have you felt your brain was in a haze or fog and you could not think clearly? Not being able to see the wood from the trees is an expression frequently used to describe that sense of being unable to think clearly. When your mind is in a haze your ability to make rational decisions is compromised and you may react or respond in a way that is not helpful to yourself or others. So how do you clear the mind? A combination of approaches is needed including healthy food choices, drinking lots of water, practicing mindfulness, meditation or other stress relieving techniques and taking regular exercise. One simple but very effective way to clear your head is to get outside in the fresh air and walk, hike, run, row, cycle, swim, garden or whatever your preferred type of activity is until you feel the fog lifting.

Try this simple exercise next time you feel the haze descending on your mind. Get outside and engage in your preferred choice of exercise or physical activity. As you move visualise the haze lifting with each step, stroke, pedal, row etc that you take. As you move picture the haze floating upwards like a cloud behind you and becoming lighter as it soars upward. Visualise it drifting across the sky, dissolving and then disappearing in the distance. Enjoy the sensation of your body moving and the lightness of your mind now that the haze has cleared. The problem or decision you are faced with will still be there but your ability to deal with it will be more effective and rational.

Exercise should be about the experience not just the outcome. Each time you engage in exercise try to focus on the physical sensation within your body. Be aware of the glands perspiring and visualise these as little detox agents cleansing your body cells. If you choose to swim, sense the lightness of your body, as it glides through the water. Swimming lengths in a pool offers the opportunity to experience a mild meditative state as you swim up and down the lanes. If you swim in the sea feel the salt water bathe your body, gently massaging it, supporting it and keeping it afloat.

Experience the sensation of letting go when you practice yoga or the buzz you feel when you are speeding down a hill on your bike or on skis. Visualise how you will feel when you complete that marathon you are training for, or the two mile hike in the woods, or that deep sea dive you have been looking forward to all week. Now go ahead and make that visualisation a reality.

Those who engage in regular exercise do so for the enjoyment of the experience as much as for the physical benefits it provides. They do not have to be convinced that being fit feels fabulous because they already know. If you are not currently a regular exerciser you have a lot to look forward to in terms of the actual experience and of course the health benefits. You will come to love being fit once you find the type of exercise that suits your personality. Many people who are non exercisers have a mental block to exercising because they associate it with working out in a gym or pounding the pavements. These forms of exercise are not for everyone, so it is important to explore what type of exercise you might enjoy and then be willing to give it a go. There is a multitude of exercise options available including hiking, running, cycling, swimming, yoga, Pilates, rowing, football, hockey, camogie, rugby, tag rugby, volleyball, basketball, badminton, tennis, martial arts, spinning, aerobics, horse riding, gymnastics, scuba diving, stand up paddling, kayaking, surfing, body boarding, rock climbing and various forms of dance, to name but a few.

Key to establishing and sustaining exercises as part of your daily routine is making sure the type of exercise you engage in has a fun element. Once exercise stops being fun your motivation will wane and before long you will start making excuses not to exercise. If you are not enjoying exercising it is time to look at an alternative form of physical activity. Try out different exercises or sports until you find the right fit for your mind and body. If you are new to exercise why not start with walking. This is the first form of exercise most of us undertook and which our bodies are designed for. Also walking requires no membership fee or specialist equipment other than a good pair of walking shoes. Get walking outdoors and see where it leads you on your wellness journey. There are many clubs, classes and groups with the common purpose of exercising together. The support of an exercise group can be fantastic when you are getting started. Not only will you enhance your physical and psychological wellness but you will also establish community connections and strengthen your social support network.

Goal setting is important when it comes to exercising. While competitive sport is not for everyone, there is something powerful in having a personal goal that motivates you to move. Motivation as we know, is the drive that energises human behaviour. Go ahead and set yourself an exercise goal and when you achieve it congratulate yourself and then set a more challenging goal to work toward. Look at our Olympians, if they did not set goals and targets they would never be in a position to compete for a medal. Do not underestimate the capacity of your body to exceed your expectations. Remember when you were a baby your body had to work hard to get moving in the first place so do not inhibit your body's ability by avoiding exercising or by setting non challenging exercise goals for yourself.

Starting today get on the road to physical fitness and reap the health and wellness benefits. You cannot avoid life challenges, but you are better equipped to deal with them when you are eating healthily, exercising regularly, practicing mindfulness and expressing gratitude. These elements combined form the basis of a wonderful lifestyle prescription that will enhance your personal wellness foundation.

Sleep Glorious Sleep

The importance of restful sleep is at times overlooked in terms of its contribution to health and wellness. The lack of adequate restful sleep impacts on your ability to function effectively in school, at work, in relationships and in all other aspects of daily life.

An average of 6-8 hours of uninterrupted sleep is essential to allow the adult body to recover and rejuvenate. Children and adolescents require more sleep than adults, to support their physical and cognitive development. However many adults and children simply do not get enough sleep. Often this is because they play computer games, engage with online media, or watch television late into the night.

Common sleep problems include, poor quality sleep, difficulty getting to sleep, restless sleep or still feeling tired in the morning. Stress and anxiety can interfere with your ability to get to sleep. The more anxious you are the less likely you are to fall asleep. This in turn can lead to further anxiety about not being able to sleep, and a vicious cycle ensues. Pain or medication may also affect your ability to get to sleep or may reduce the quality or duration of your sleep. If pain or medication is affecting your sleep patterns you should speak with your doctor, to have the underlying cause identified and addressed.

Each person is different and the amount of sleep you require varies throughout your life. Babies and young children need a lot more sleep than adults, so it is important to establish a bed time routine that promotes restful sleep. Teenagers also need a lot of sleep because their bodies are undergoing rapid growth and development. If your teenager seems to be sleeping a lot more than you think is natural, they are not being lazy; they are merely listening to their bodies. Of course if your teenager is staying up late at night and is exhausted in the morning, that is an entirely different matter.

We need to recognise the important role of sleep in supporting physical and mental health at all stages of life and take practical steps to ensure that we and those we care for get ample high quality sleep. One way to do so is to minimise the use of technology prior to going to bed. The brain is very active when we are engaged with technology and to expect it to automatically switch to sleep mode is unrealistic. Aim to avoid the use of technology for at least one to two hours before going to bed and make this longer for children. This means switching off the television, phone, computers or whatever technology you are using that may interfere with restful sleep. Remove these gadgets from your bedroom so as to resist the temptation to check messages or emails when you hear the *ping* of an incoming alert during the night.

Your sleep environment impacts on the quality of sleep. A cluttered or noisy environment is not conducive to restful sleep. We place a high value on ensuring babies and small children get plenty of undisturbed sleep, by keeping their sleeping environment calm and distraction free. Why then would we have a different approach for older children and adults? Your bedroom should be conducive to restful sleep, so air the room every day and aim to keep it clutter and noise free, when you are sleeping.

Other ways to promote restful sleep include establishing a bedtime routine for your children and yourself; taking regular exercise outdoors; avoiding caffeine or other stimulants after seven o'clock in the evening and eating a healthy diet. You can also use heavy curtains or blinds to avoid too much light entering the bedroom as this can disturb your sleep cycle. Room temperature is a factor in restful sleep so maintain a stable room temperature during the night. Aim also to relax before retiring to bed, perhaps by listening to soothing music, meditating or having a warm bath. Try to avoid arguments before bedtime as it will upset you and this will disrupt your sleep. If you do have an argument you should try to resolve it before going to bed. Alternatively agree to discuss the matter in the morning instead of arguing at bedtime. This may be a difficult ask, but in the light of day you may view things differently.

The Steering Wheel of Your Life

We know that our physical body is the perfect vehicle to carry us as we journey through life but we also need to cultivate a well mind. Mental wellness incorporates your emotional and psychological wellness. These building blocks of wellness interact with your physical and spiritual wellness and if one block is out of sync it affects other aspects your life. A common barrier to mental wellness is a lack of confidence and self esteem. If you have low self esteem you may instinctively seek out unhealthy relationships because you do not believe that you deserve to be treated with love, care and respect. Unhealthy relationships further reinforce your low self esteem, particularly if you experience abuse within the relationship.

When you experience emotional pain or you have low self esteem, you may engage in self defeating practices such as isolating yourself from others or, avoiding social situations. Although you may need support to process how you are feeling, you may be too afraid or ashamed to ask for help. Low self esteem often results in having limited expectations for one's life. If you do not feel deserving of success in your life, you may unknowingly sabotage your opportunities for personal achievements.

Some people with low self esteem feel victimised and seek to blame others for their personal circumstances. Others become like stage actors and go through life wearing a mask that portrays an image that everything is fine. Such a mask disguises the person's emotional pain, and by wearing a mask the person is denying their inner truth which negates against their mental and spiritual wellness. If you lack self esteem you may have surrendered your personal power and it can feel like someone else is in the driving seat of your life.

Close your eyes for a moment and visualise yourself in the back seat of a beautiful car. There is someone in the driving seat who seems familiar but you cannot figure out where you know them from. You have not yet recognized the driver as your doubting self, whose actions are fuelled by fear. Having spent some time revving the engine of your beautiful car the driver takes off at high speed and you feel powerless. You start to cry out but the driver shouts at you to be quiet and tells you that they are in charge. You do as you are told because you do not have the confidence to stand up for yourself. You hold on for dear life as they continue at high speed. You feel physically sick and mentally paralysed.

Suddenly the car turns off the road and heads for a cliff edge. You know that if the driver does not stop, the car will go over the edge and you may die. From deep inside your voice of personal power rises up and shouts "stop". Immediately the driver hits the brakes and the car comes to a sudden stop within a few feet of the cliff edge. Even though you are shaking you step out, open the door on the driver's side and muster up the courage to tell the driver to get out. They refuse but you become assertive and explain in no uncertain terms that they are not welcome in your car and will never again take over the steering wheel of your life. They reluctantly leave and for a while you can hear the sound of their angry voice criticising you from a distance. As you take some deep cleansing breaths their voice disappears and silence is restored. You tell yourself that you can drive this car home and although you feel nervous you get home safe and well and feel a huge sense pride and relief.

When you reflect on what has just happened you begin to realise that you did not have the confidence to take control of the steering wheel of your own life. Instead you surrendered personal power to the shadow side of you which is fuelled by fear, emotional pain and anxiety. This experience taught you a valuable lesson; namely that if you surrender to fear, emotional pain and the voice of the negative inner commentator it can paralyse you and undermine your personal wellness foundation.

This is a scenario that you might see in a movie but in many ways your life is like a movie with you as the main actor. Are you the victim in the movie of your life or are you the hero or heroine. Victims tend to have low self esteem and lack the confidence to stand up for their beliefs and assert their personal power and truth. Typically in the movie the victim is transformed into the hero or heroine and in the fairy tale they live happily ever after. You too can have your happy ever after because it is you who is in charge of your life choices from this moment onwards. To reclaim control you need to dismantle the barriers to your mental and emotional wellness and take back control of the steering wheel of your life.

Releasing Stress and Restoring Balance

Unhealthy levels of stress have become a significant factor in modern society and stress has emerged in recent years as a precursor to many chronic diseases and mental health difficulties. Positive stress is linked to new experiences, facing up to challenges, building on your strengths and increasing your coping abilities. If you try to avoid stress by staying in what you consider to be a safe place you will never be challenged and your life will become mundane. You will lose your motivation for new learning or adventure and may end up seeking comfort or pleasure from food, television, online media, alcohol or other sources of artificial pleasure or enjoyment. This only serves to create an imbalance in your body which can lead to further physical or emotional stress or in some cases ill health.

Perception is a key factor when it comes to stress. If you are faced with a situation or a demand that you perceive as being too much to cope with, chances are you will feel stressed about it. Everyone has a certain amount of stress in their life and some are better able to cope than others. Stress is fine as long as it does not move to a level where it causes distress. It becomes a problem when you feel you can no longer cope and become overwhelmed. This is negative stress and is often underpinned by fear. Perhaps you have a fear of the unknown, a fear of making the wrong decision, a fear of what others will think about you or a fear that you do not have the skills or ability to deal with a particular situation or challenge. Often your negative inner commentator is fuelling this fear. Fear can be paralysing and you may become stuck in a fear based state of stress where you feel powerless to change your situation.

When faced with high levels of stress you can lose sight of the power of your marvellous body to restore balance and harmony. Your physical body is your partner in managing stress but you need to work with it, not against it. Your body is constantly working to regulate your breathing, heart rate, hormones, temperature, digestion, sleep, cell repair and all the other physiological functions it undertakes on a daily basis. You owe it to your body to support it in its efforts to maintain balance and this includes controlling stress. If your diet is unhealthy, or you are consuming excess alcohol, or you are not physically active, or you are getting too little sleep, then your risk factors for physiological stress are increased and you are working against your body instead of with it.

Hormones are chemical messengers that tell different cells of the body how to behave. The human body is well equipped to regulate hormone levels in order to maintain internal physiological balance. Two hormones in particular are produced to deal with stress, namely adrenaline and cortisol. Adrenaline is the hormone that quickly prepares the body for fight or flight when faced with a sudden stressful situation. Cortisol, also known as the stress hormone has a delayed secretion after a stressful event and helps the body deal with ongoing stress. A problem arises when you have a continued release of cortisol, because you are at risk of developing adrenal fatigue. Common features of adrenal fatigue include feeling tired for no obvious reason, constantly feeling rundown or overwhelmed, having difficulty recovering from minor illness, craving salty and sweet snacks on an ongoing basis and feeling more awake, alert and energetic after six in the evening than you do all day. If you have experienced a number of these symptoms you should consult your doctor to have a medical check up. You might also consider making an appointment with a nutritionist to see if any aspects of your diet are contributing to your symptoms.

When stress has taken control of your life an imbalance has occurred between mindfulness and busyness. This imbalance moves you away from wellness and toward dis-ease and illness. The less mindful you are the busier you may feel, but ironically, your productivity is likely to be reduced. You strive to find control in your life but the more you attempt to control events the less power you have. It becomes a vicious cycle because, the less control you feel you have, the more you try to take control. You lose perspective and begin to associate personal power with being in control. In truth however personal power comes from letting go of the need to be in control.

Imagine it is a windy day and you are in an enclosed park, with a deep pond and tall trees. A man drives his truck into the park, gets out, goes to the back of the truck and opens the rear door. As he opens the door, balloons start to float out and a sudden gust of wind whips them upwards. The driver looks around anxiously to see who can help. He asks you to assist him retrieve the balloons and to put them back in the truck. Without giving it any thought you set about trying to catch the balloons. The wind has blown some of them into the pond, others have got stuck in the branches of the trees and more are floating up and over the railings surrounding the park. You can see them drifting off in the distance and you know there is no hope of catching them. A few balloons are blowing around the grounds of the park so you try to collect these. As you get close to each one a gust of wind catches it and blows it further away from you.

You finally manage to catch one balloon. You continue to try to catch another balloon for the next few minutes. You find yourself getting increasingly frustrated and you are starting to feel annoyed and stressed. Under your breath you scream at the wind to stop blowing, you curse the balloons for being so light, you are irritated at the city council for putting trees and a pond in the park, and you wonder what sort of a foolish person, would release balloons on a windy day.

You are now standing in the middle of the park holding one balloon feeling irritated and annoyed at the truck driver. A lady who has been sitting on a park bench watching you asks you what you are doing. Tempted to say "what does it look like" you instead grit your teeth and tell her you are trying to catch the balloons and put them back in the truck. She looks at you as you stand there with the one balloon in your hand and asks this simple question.

"For what purpose are you doing this?" You have no answer. You have been busy chasing balloons on a windy day without thinking about it. A little child passes by with her mother and you hand her the balloon.

You leave the park annoyed with yourself but a little wiser. You have learned the valuable lesson that some things are outside of your control (in this case the wind, the pond, the trees and the height of the railings) but that you have control over your thoughts and actions. You resolve to stop and ask the question "for what purpose?" the next time you are faced with a difficult decision or a request from someone else for action.

Okay so this is an exaggerated example of loss of mindfulness, but think about it for a moment. How many times every day do you find yourself rushing from one task to the next, responding to demands from others and ending up feeling stressed and exhausted. Are you living your life trying to catch balloons in the wind? You need to stop when you feel like this and ask yourself "for what purpose am I doing this?" If you do not stop to reflect on your actions, you are at risk of burn out, and you will end up stressed and with little balance in your life. It is time to release stress and reclaim balance in your life. You can start today by taking the air out of the balloons of anxiety and worry and start to practice mindfulness.

From Busyness to Mindfulness

We are living in a world that pressures us to rush through living and in doing so bypass the present moments of our lives. Motorways and bypasses have been built around villages, towns and cities to speed up traffic flow and to reduce congestion. This makes practical sense if a driver needs to get from point A to point B within a specific timeframe. Our life journey starts at point A which is the first *breath* and ends at the Z point called *death*. Every living moment between breath and death really matters and should be embraced and enjoyed. If we want to appreciate our personal life journey we have to get off the motorway and enjoy the scenic route without wishing we were somewhere else. There is nothing wrong with taking time out of our hurried lives to have a picnic, to take a walk along a river bank, to dip your toes in the sea or lake, to dance in the moon light, to build sandcastles or to make snow angels. We need to become mindful in how we live our lives because when we get to the inevitable death point of our journey it would be a pity to have missed the opportunities presented along the way, because we were too busy bypassing the present moment.

A starting point for mindfulness is becoming aware of your breath. Your life journey is aligned with the first breath you take and ends when you take your last breath and your physical body dies. This in effect means that we are only ever one breath away from death, but we do not know which breath will be our last. With this in mind we should value every breath we get to take. As you inhale each new breath you are welcoming life into your body, and as you release the out breath you are letting go that which the body and mind does not require. This makes breathing a form of deep cleansing for the mind, body and spirit.

Visualise the out breath as a waterfall, with all the stress, tension and anxiety flowing away never to return. Your next out breath will never be drawn in again and your next in breath will not include what was just released. A waterfall cascading down the side of a mountain carries with it water and other deposits that are dispersed in the pool below. Water will never flow down that waterfall again in the same order or composition, no matter how long the waterfall exists. This is also the case with your out breath.

On each out breath you have the opportunity to release the emotional and psychological baggage that has been weighing heavy on your mind and eroding your personal power to steer your own life course. Practice letting go of this baggage as you exhale, and as you inhale, visualise your body and mind filling up with the personal power that will enable you to deal with your life challenges. In any meditation or mindfulness practice it always comes back to your breath, because breath is the font of life. Bless your breath and breathe toward wellness.

For some people, prayer is a form of meditation and it helps them achieve inner peace, acceptance and serenity in their lives. For others, connecting with nature supports mindfulness and helps them to release stress. Nature is in perfect balance and harmony, so being close to nature can support you in restoring balance in your life.

More formal meditation and mindfulness practices have become increasingly popular, as way of releasing stress and finding peace. The practice of regular meditation and mindfulness is having a positive impact on universal wellness, and should be strengthened and actively encouraged.

Aside from breath work and meditation there are many other practices that promote physical, emotional and spiritual wellness and which may help you manage stress and achieve balance in your life. Some of these include Emotional Freedom Technique or Tapping as it more commonly referred to. Tapping can be particularly beneficial if you are feeling anxious about an important decision or an upcoming potentially stressful event. It is a simple, but very effective technique for letting go of that which is hindering you from achieving your full potential.

Other therapies and techniques that have been around for a while involve changing your thought process, behaviours and associations and include among others, Neuro Linguistic Programming, Cognitive Behaviour Therapy and Brief Intervention Therapy. There are also a range of complimentary therapies that can help you control stress in your life, restore balance and support your personal healing and inner wellness. Some of these include aromatherapy, homeopathy, reflexology, reiki, bio-energy healing and massage.

Irrespective of what technique or therapies you choose you have to realise that on its own it will not eliminate stress or restore balance in your life. Wellness is a whole person approach so you also need to address other lifestyle factors including your diet, exercise, sleep and your relationship with yourself and others.

A Daily Dose of Laughter

Laughter is a powerful antidote to stress, is absolutely free and has tangible benefits in terms of mental and physical health. It is impossible to feel sad while you are laughing. Unfortunately in modern life many people seem to have forgotten how to laugh, or it may be a long time since they have had a decent laugh. We are bombarded on a daily basis with negative news stories about the economy, political conflict, war, murder or another human tragedy somewhere in the world. It seems as though there is very little to laugh about in modern society. The sound of an adult laughing is a rare event and pessimism has become the default position for many. Our bodies, minds and spirits are not experiencing regular fun and laughter which is a pity, because laughter is a great tension and stress reliever. There is an old saying that laughter is the best medicine, but many adults almost express an apology if they are seen to be laughing when the world is in such a sorry state. It is frightening to think that something that comes so natural has become so rare. Are we extinguishing our spirit of fun and if so where is the joy and happiness going to come from or how is it going to be expressed?

Children on the other hand do not restrain their sense of fun and if you pass a school yard or playground you will hear the joyous peals of childhood laughter. Children have not been contaminated with the dark cloud of gloom that many adults appear to be weighed down by. Unless we change our mindset and find silver linings on these clouds we will silence the laughter of our children and the positive energy that comes from joy and laughter will fade.

Laughter if it were a universal lifestyle prescription might read something like this. Have three laughs a day, morning, afternoon and in the evening, and repeat each time you feel angry, sad, stressed or upset. We should not have to prescribe laughter but sometimes people need reminding of the importance of laughter to their mental health and wellness. Laughter should be as much a part of your daily diet as is food and water. The absence of fun and laughter in your life is a barrier to mental, physical and spiritual wellness so we need to get back on the laughter trail.

It is time to give expression to the comedian within. It was always there but might have got suppressed by the imposed seriousness of life. Your challenge, if you accept it, is to dig deep, unearth your laugh and cultivate it until it is blooming again.

There are numerous ways to bring laughter into your life, including, going to a comedy show, watching a funny movie, telling jokes, rolling down a grassy hill, playing hopscotch just as you did when you were a child, reading a funny story, letting your child tickle you, going roller skating or trying a sport or activity you have never tried before. The secret is to give yourself permission to laugh if you fall over or trip up.

Once you bring laughter back into your life you will crave more of it. This is a good craving, so feed it and continuously satisfy it. Set yourself free, let your hair down, have fun and enjoy yourself. The only person you need permission from to laugh is you. So, from today onwards say yes to laughter. Trust me you will feel better, your emotional wellness will blossom, you will be less stressed and your life satisfaction will increase. That gives you a lot to smile about so from this moment onwards start medicating your life with laughter.

The Working Well

After family, school is the next community the child becomes a member of. If children struggle in the school environment they may struggle when they move to the wider learning community of college and the workplace. If a child is not stimulated in accordance with their ability they will regress or fail to progress intellectually or academically while in school. Likewise if they are challenged beyond their ability the same will happen and their experience of school may not be a happy or satisfying one. Equally if a college student is studying a course that they have no real interest in, or which they find academically too challenging, they will either drop out or struggle through until the end of the course. They may end up with a qualification in an area for which they have no interest in pursuing a career. This affects not only their psychological and emotional wellness but also their future occupational opportunities.

Every child has different interests, learning needs and abilities and the formal education system cannot provide a bespoke curriculum for every student. However if education is holistic by design it will support the physical, psychological, emotional and spiritual wellness of each student. With increasing cutbacks in education budgets, schools are faced with reductions to the learning supports and resources required by some students. As a result many are left to navigate their way through an education system that is primarily focussed on academic outcomes. It is important to remind ourselves that if we value wellness then we must support all children to achieve their full potential in all aspects of their life. We can start by challenging the educational barriers that currently exist. We must powerfully advocate for education systems that support the wellness, of every child on this planet. Each child deserves to be empowered through education and training, to achieve their full potential in all aspects of their lives.

As we move beyond education we find that barriers to occupational wellness also exist for adults. For many people work is a source of income and provides them with a sense of purpose and a valued role in society. Unemployment, underemployment, lack of job security, dependence on social welfare payments, low wages, job dissatisfaction, negative work cultures, workplace inequality, lack of recognition for work undertaken, work overload, lack of promotional opportunities or feeling trapped in a job you do not enjoy all impact on your mental and physical wellness.

Aside from financial commitments most people want to engage in a meaningful occupation that they enjoy and from which they derive satisfaction. If the occupation you are engaged in does not match your interests, preferences and values you will not enjoy it and may even dread the thought of going to work each day. If you are unhappy in your work it will affect your mental wellness which may in turn affect your performance. This is a vicious circle because if your performance is below standard this will affect your promotion opportunities.

The workplace culture can support positive health and wellness, or conversely, if employees are not valued and respected it can contribute to dis-ease and stress. Many workplaces have policies aimed at preventing discrimination and promoting equality, and these are implemented in a manner that encourages employees to raise concerns. Other workplaces however, tolerate discrimination or inequitable practices. If an employee has little job security they may be reluctant to raise concerns, or to challenge such a culture.

For some workers, low wages, long hours and a lack of positive recognition leaves them feeling undervalued and disillusioned. This inhibits wellness in the workplace and leads to anxiety, dissatisfaction and in many cases work related stress, which spills over into other aspects of the persons' life.

Workplace wellness is not just about workload, it also includes the psychological and social environment of the workplace. Managers and colleagues all contribute to this environment. Many employers have recognised the importance of wellness within the workplace and promote a culture where employees are valued and where concerns and complaints are dealt with promptly. Some workplaces have introduced employee wellness programmes because they recognise that well employees have greater job satisfaction, are likely to be happier at work and in turn will be more productive. By investing in employee wellness programmes including offering wellness and health coaching, the employer gets the return on the investment through reduced absenteeism, increased productivity and in some cases higher profits. Not every organisation or company will have a workplace wellness programme and where one is available not every employee will avail of it. This reflects the choice each individual makes in respect of their personal wellness at work.

You can resent others for what they have or have not done in the workplace, or alternatively you can seek ways of making your work more meaningful and satisfying. Practical steps to improve your occupational wellness include identifying your dream job or occupation and determining what changes you need to make in order to fulfil this. Your dream should include the type of work you would like to be involved in and the reasons why this interests you. This may be paid or unpaid but should reflect your passions and interests. Perhaps you are unemployed but would like to start your own business, if so write down in detail the type of business you would like to have.

Follow the same approach if you are in business but would like to do something different; or if you would like to change jobs or career; or if you would like to become a volunteer; or if you would like to re-train or go back to education; or if you would like to quit your job and be a homemaker; or if you would like to start making crafts; or if you would like to join a farmers market or, whatever your preferred occupation is.

When you start to identify your dream occupation it is probable that you will come up with factors that may impact on your ability to achieve this. Some of these may include fear of rejection or ridicule, lack of relevant education, training or experience, or your current financial commitments or family responsibilities. These may seem like obstacles now but there is no reason why you cannot overcome these one by one in order to fulfil your work related dreams and ambition. Your dream is the starting point and you will later need to develop a plan to make this happen. The planning process will include setting goals and timeframes to achieve your dream and identifying the resources and supports you need to help you succeed.

Writing a book has been an ambition of mine for many years but up until recently I had not committed to it nor had I taken action to make it happen. When I was ready to start translating my ambition into reality I started off by developing a plan. This involved setting goals for completing the writing phase of the project and linking in with the resources and support available to me. I set targets for myself in relation to how many words I wanted to have written by certain dates and this helped keep me focused and on track.

When it comes to your dreams, ambitions and goals be true to yourself and commit to making them a reality. You can achieve your true potential and experience fulfilment in your life's work but it starts with you. Let today be the beginning of your occupational wellness journey and do not let anyone block your path to personal satisfaction and fulfilment.

PART SIX
Next Steps on Your Personal Life Journey

Growing Your Personal Wellness Foundation

I hope that some of the guidance I have offered in this book will support you in continuing to build your personal wellness foundation and harvest your inner wisdom. Before we finish I want to share with you some practical steps you can take to prioritise wellness in your life. These steps are based on a combination of the personal centered quality of life model I developed, and the Real Balance Wellness Mapping 360° Methodology™ developed by Dr Michael Arloski, author of *Wellness Coaching for Lasting Lifestyle Change*.

In taking the next steps on your well life journey, I encourage you to surround yourself with trusted allies, who will support you as you make the choices and changes necessary to blossom in wellness and wisdom. You might consider engaging a Wellness Coach who will guide and support you to reclaim your personal power and take control of the steering wheel of your life.

Many people go through life never quite figuring out what their life purpose is and as a result they fail to live a satisfying life. If you are experiencing a lot of negativity, dissatisfaction or unhappiness in your life then perhaps you are not living in accordance with your personal values, beliefs and your inner truth. Have you ever found yourself asking the following questions? "What is it all about?" or "is this all there is to my life?" or "surely there must be a better life?" or saying to yourself "I am sick and tired of living like this!"

If so then your personal wellness foundation needs some attention. Now is the right time to examine if your patterns of behaviour and lifestyle choices are supporting your wellness and life satisfaction. If what you have been doing up to now is no longer working for you in terms of your quality of life then something needs to change.

Building your personal wellness foundation requires you to first identify what changes you wish to make in your life and then to take the practical steps necessary to make these changes. Making any change including those related to diet, exercise, stress, education, your occupation, relationships, community participation or spiritual practice will present some challenges but also many opportunities. The key is to determine what changes you want to make, and how ready, willing and committed you are to make these changes a reality. The level of passion you have in relation to your desired change is a significant factor in determining how ready you are to take action. If you are passionate about improving your health and wellness this is a plus in getting you off the blocks and onto the wellness track.

Important also is the extent to which you believe that you are responsible for your health and wellness, and that you are capable of making whatever changes are necessary to improve your quality of life. If you do not own your personal power then you may seek to blame others when you do not succeed, or you may start making excuses when you are struggling to implement a change in your life. Once you start down the route of blaming others or making excuses, you are giving ammunition to the negative inner commentator and self doubt will creep in. Your thoughts and your attitude can either support or sabotage your efforts, so it is important to be aware of these and consider if they are helping or hindering you to improve your quality of life. If you find yourself coming up with excuses then you have not yet taken full responsibility for your health and wellness and an attitude adjustment maybe required.

Your capacity to change is based on a number of factors including your level of self belief, your self esteem, the resources, supports and opportunities available to you, your personal circumstances and your past experiences. But the most important factor is how much you really want to make changes in your life. When I played football our coaches often said to us before a game, that if we wanted to win the game we had to be hungry for success. Simply, because half hearted efforts do not win trophies. This proved to be true in terms of our track record. Those times when we were literally starving for a win were the days when we pulled out every stop and never gave up until the final whistle. If we did not win the game we would of course be disappointed but could walk away proud of our individual and collective team efforts. Games like these always made us better players because we stretched ourselves beyond mediocrity toward excellence.

You have to become hungry for wellness of mind, body and spirit and then be whole hearted in your efforts to do whatever it takes to live a well and fulfilling life. You are not necessarily going to achieve every goal or implement every change in the timeframe you want, but it is better to be on the path to personal wellness than to be a couch spectator. It is okay not to achieve every goal but it is not okay to give up on your dreams and vision for a better quality of life. If you find yourself drifting away from your path to wellness, then it is time to reach out for support. The supports available to you may be physical, emotional, social, material, civic or environmental in nature. Their availability combined with your willingness to access them will influence the extent to which you take action to improve your life or lifestyle. A Wellness Coach can help you get back on track and stay focussed on your dreams and life goals, and will be your ally as you journey toward wellness and wisdom.

Another key factor in determining if you will make changes in your life is your perception of the benefits these changes will have on your quality of life. If you believe that you are capable of changing how you live your life and you recognise the long term benefits, then you are more likely to commit to and stick with the change. If you lack confidence in your ability to make changes in your life then a "fake it until you make it" or "can do" attitude can be helpful in getting you started. Once you are ready the only thing that can get in your way of making changes to improve your life, is you.

A useful starting point in building your personal wellness foundation is to establish your satisfaction with your current quality of life including your health and wellness. You may feel dissatisfied with aspects of your life but it is important to take time out to examine what is working well for you and what aspects of your life you want to improve. When things are not working well in some aspects of your life this can impact on your overall sense of wellness, and you can quickly lose sight of all that is good in your life. I suggest that you take an A4 sheet of paper or open up a word document on your computer and divide it into two columns. The first column is for all the things that you are satisfied with in your life. Try to fill this first column from the top to the bottom of the page, with a list of everything you can think of that is positive or working well in your life.

What you list is totally personal but for some it may include having an income, being able to hear music and birdsong, having the gift of friendship, the health of your children or family, having kind neighbours, the beauty of nature, your child being happy in school or at work, an illness being in remission, being free to make your own life choices, being in a loving relationship or if you are single perhaps enjoying your personal space. It does not matter what is on your list as long as you take the time to examine and acknowledge all the things in your life that are satisfying or working well.

The second column is for the things that are not working well or aspects of your life that you are not satisfied with. Do not however, give into the temptation to start filling this column until you have the first column completed. The reason for this is that we human beings tend to find it easier to list our problems than to list the positives in our lives. When you focus on the negative aspects of your life or lifestyle, the negative inner commentator jumps into action, and *'stinking thinking* begins. By the time your negative list is complete you will feel despondent and less able to focus on all that is good in your life. However if you start with what is working well and record these in the first column, your frame of mind is going to be more affirmative and you can look at the things that are not working well more objectively.

When both columns are complete look at your lists to see if there is an imbalance between the things you are satisfied with and those with which you are dissatisfied. There is seldom a 50-50 split and at different times and for different reasons your satisfaction with various aspects of your life will change. However if there is an ongoing imbalance between what you perceive to be working well and what is not working well, you need to work on restoring some balance.

From a Dream to a Vision

When you have identified your current level of life satisfaction it is important that you identify those aspects of your life that you are happy to maintain and those areas that you want to address. This can be challenging and you may feel overwhelmed by the list of things you feel you need to change. A starting point is getting clear on what it is that you want to achieve in your life and Dr Michael Arloski (1997) refers to this as your "Life Vision."

Over the years you may have made New Year resolutions or set goals related to diet, exercise, quitting smoking, reducing alcohol consumption, career or occupation, relationships, hobbies, finances, holidays or home. You may have achieved some of these but perhaps not all, for various reasons. Irrespective of what your resolutions or goals were or are, a common denominator for most people is the desire to make changes in how they live their life. Ultimately change it is about achieving greater life satisfaction and personal fulfilment, but most people do not think about it in this way, nor do they give much thought as to why a particular change is important.

Many of those who struggle to make and sustain changes in their life end up telling themselves that it is not worth the effort, and unfortunately they give up on their personal dreams or goals. Had they given sufficient thought as to why they should bother with the change in the first place, they would have a clearer vision of what their life will be like when they make the change and achieve their goals. When you give up on your dreams you end up with low levels of life satisfaction. If you are serious about building the foundation for a better quality of life it is important to develop a clear vision of what you want to achieve and how you want to live your life. This may require some initial dream building from which you can then clarify your vision for your life. You can write down your vision for your life, type it on your computer, make a digital recording of it or, if you are artistic capture it in a drawing or painting.

If you digitally record your life vision save it on your mobile device and play it back anytime you are starting to doubt your ability to make changes in your life. If you create a picture of your life vision, display it somewhere prominent where you will see it every day. This way it becomes a constant reminder of where you are heading on your life journey. If you write it down read it every morning and every night so it becomes the focus of your day and is imprinted in your mind before you go to sleep. If it is on your personal computer use it as your screen saver so you are reminded of it every time you log on. The important thing is to own your life vision, let it reflect your truth, let your life choices be guided by it and never allow anyone else to dismiss it or trample on it. As you continue on your life journey your vision will evolve to reflect your changing circumstances and your emerging personal dreams, hopes and aspirations.

Some of you may struggle initially to articulate your life vision and it may seem like a self indulgent exercise, and others may feel guilty about spending time on this type of personal work. If you have not been encouraged in the past to set goals or if you have never done anything like this before you may need the support of a Wellness Coach or a trusted friend to get started. Your vision for your life becomes the blueprint for how you choose to live from here onwards so it is important not to rush the process. Imagine it being similar to building a house. A house design starts with a vision of what it will look like and then the architect draws up the plans. When these are agreed the building work begins. You are the architect of your own life so invest in developing your vision and then design a plan to make this vision a reality.

It is important to set aside some quiet time for this work where you will not be disturbed. You need a clear head and a stress free environment to give it your full attention. There is little point trying to develop a vision for your life if the television or radio is blaring, or the children are demanding your attention, or if you are under time pressure. You need to feel relaxed with an open mind and heart because this is one of the most important things you can do for yourself. Find a quiet space to start the dream building process. Some of you may choose to go for a walk on a quiet beach, or along a river bank or take a hike in the hills or woods to clear your mind of the chatter of everyday life. Others may be content to sit in their garden or at the kitchen table. The key is to find a place where you feel comfortable, relaxed and open to envisioning your desired life and lifestyle.

Reflection is an important element in creating your life vision as it can bring clarity to your thoughts. It is worthwhile reflecting on your life so far to determine what you have learned, what has worked well for you, what you have enjoyed, what has not worked well for you, who have been the most influential people in your life, when in your life have you felt content, happy or fulfilled and what was happening at that point in time that contributed to those feelings. Some of you may have had a great sense of achievement when you were involved in sports, or drama or volunteering or studying or playing music or parenting or while engaging in a particular job or hobby. Others may have felt a deep sense of calm when they practiced yoga, meditated, walked on a beach, painted, cooked, knitted, went horse riding or went fishing. It does not matter what the activity was, rather, it is the experience and enjoyment of the activity that is important. It may not be possible to engage in the same activity again but there will be other things you can try that would produce a similar feeling or sense of enjoyment. You will not know until your try.

I used to scuba dive a number of years ago and there is a lot of preparation before a dive. The diving gear is heavy and a lot of time is spent assembling and disassembling equipment and carrying out safety checks before and after every dive. However the benefits far outweigh the effort involved. Once you are under the water you are transported to a magical world. The peace and silence combined with the anticipation of what you might see or find in such beautiful surroundings is invigorating. Every dive is different in terms of marine life but on every dive you experience a feeling of freedom and a sense of being at one with nature. I can no longer scuba dive but am still able to go swimming and snorkelling which although not the same as diving, is none the less a thoroughly enjoyable experience in the water.

So even if you are no longer able to engage in an activity that previously brought you enjoyment and a sense of wellness this does not mean you cannot experience these feelings again. You just need to broaden your horizons and be open to new experiences. Remember you have the power to choose and the freedom to dream. Let your life vision reflect your dreams and aspirations, and let it reveal your inner truth. Make it a reality and enjoy an exciting personal journey toward fulfilling your vision and life purpose.

From Vision to Reality

Your dreams and life vision should excite you and you should be passionate about making them a reality. If you are not excited about the changes you want to make you are going to lose your motivation when the going gets tough. Harness your excitement and passion into an energy force and start working on designing your personal wellness plan to translate your vision into reality.

The old saying "Rome was not built in a day" is true in terms of your life vision and personal wellness plan. There may be a number of things you want to achieve in life but it may not be realistic to try to accomplish all of these at once. Some may be things you want to address immediately and others may be less urgent so can be left for another time. However you should set a time frame for each aspect of your life vision as otherwise it may be sidelined, or procrastination may set in.

The key to developing a personal wellness plan or as Dr Michael Arloski (1997) describes it your *Wellness Map,* is being specific about what you want to achieve, what changes you want to make and when and how are you going to make this happen. For example if you have said in your life vision you want to lose weight and get fit this will involve change in two areas of your life, namely diet and exercise. There will be overlaps between these areas but it is important to identify specific goals for each one. A sample goal might be to lose five kilograms in weight and go down one dress size. This now becomes your goal in relation to diet but you also need to set a specific timeframe by which you want to have achieved this goal. Keep the goals realistic and attainable otherwise you are setting yourself up for failure.

Once you have identified your goals you need to identify the action steps you will take to achieve these. In identifying the action steps consider the resources and supports you will need, and the current commitments you have that might impact on your ability to complete these. For example if you want to change jobs but you are not in a position to do so in the short term due to family commitments, this does not mean you should give up on this goal. Rather you could identify the steps you can take to set the wheels in motion in order to change your job within a specific timeframe. This might involve updating your curriculum vitae, or undertaking a training course to give you the skills or qualification for the particular job you would like to be doing. Your life vision and goals create the blueprint for your well life journey and should not be set aside because there are some factors preventing you from achieving everything in the short term.

When you are designing your personal wellness plan think about how ready you are to take the necessary actions to implement your plan. Some people I coach are very enthusiastic about goal setting and creating a list of the actions they are going to take to achieve their goals. However many find it difficult to get off the starting blocks because they are not yet ready to leap into action. There is a big difference between wanting to do something and being ready to do something. This is where goals can be broken down into small actions steps which are doable. For example you may want to cut down on your caffeine consumption because you currently drink six cups of coffee a day and this is impacting on your sleep and concentration. Although you are not ready to give up coffee completely an action to help reduce your consumption would be to swap your evening cup of coffee for a cup of decaffeinated coffee, herbal tea or water. Gradually you can work toward replacing all your cups of coffee with decaffeinated coffee, herbal tea or water. I am a great believer in one small swap at a time as a starting point for making changes in your life and lifestyle. If you swap one biscuit a day for one piece of fruit, or one coffee for one cup of herbal tea, or one half hour in front of the television for one thirty minute walk you are gently building change into your life which has an increased likelihood of being sustained, and which you can build on over time.

A key factor but one that is sometimes overlooked in terms of your success in achieving your goals is your willingness to reach out for support. To minimise the risk of relapse or giving up on your vision and goals it is important to identify what supports you can tap into. Who are the people in your life who will encourage and support you to implement your personal wellness plan? The supports available to you may be determined by a range of factors including your relationship with the people in your life, your geographic location, your financial situation, your access to child care and transport or your access to technology including the internet. Some of the supports or resources you might tap into include family, friends, work colleagues, professionals such as a dietician or nutritionist, a holistic therapist, your medical practitioner, a counsellor, a career guidance officer, a fitness instructor, a health and wellness coach, a career, business or life coach, a support group, a sports or leisure club, online forums, education programmes, your church or your local library. As you design your personal wellness plan ensure you identify what supports you will need and how and when you will access these.

Dr Michael Arloski (1997) reinforces the importance of evaluating and reviewing your progress as you implement changes in your life. We move forward when we achieve our goals so the importance of reviewing how you are progressing in relation to your vision and goals cannot be under estimated. The only way to know if you have achieved your goals and if you are fulfilling your life vision is by reviewing on a regular basis how you are getting on with your actions.

There are numerous ways you can record and evaluate how your personal wellness plan is progressing but the method you use must suit your personality. If you love technology then computer applications for monitoring and recording your physical activity, food intake or other lifestyle behaviours may work well for you. For someone else, an electronic or paper based calendar, diary or journal may be a preferred method for recording when actions or goals have been completed. Others may prefer to write a blog or use an online tracking tool. Others may commit to ringing their Wellness Coach, a friend or a member of their support group to give an update on their progress. Irrespective of which method you choose it should be simple to use and should provide evidence of your achievements.

Monitoring and evaluating your progress gives recognition to your achievements, and provides an early indicator of when you are starting to go off track. If you are not monitoring your progress and evaluating where you are at in relation to your goals you may be kidding yourself about what you have eaten, how much exercise you have taken, how much study you have completed, how many words you have written on that assignment or novel, or how many times this week you practiced breath work or meditated.

If you find yourself slipping off track or making excuses for why you are not implementing your goals then you need to identify what is interfering with your plan. In the early days of change the risk of giving up exists. As you evaluate what went wrong you may find that you did not sustain the changes because you were not committed to, or ready to make the change, or you did not seek the support you needed at the outset. In life there is no certainty and an unexpected life event can dramatically change your circumstances and impact on your ability to implement your goals. It is therefore important to review your life vision and personal wellness plan at regular intervals particularly when there has been a significant change in your personal life circumstances.

You are on an evolving journey of personal growth and development and what may have been a priority a few months ago, or last year may seem less important today. Inevitably however as you grow in wellness and wisdom other priorities will emerge, and as they do add them to your vision and personal wellness plan. Review your progress, revisit your goals, link into the supports available to you and most importantly never lose sight of your vision for wellness, personal life satisfaction, happiness and fulfilment. Stay on track in implementing your personal wellness plan by tapping into your personal resilience, creativity and resourcefulness and then harness the external supports and resources available to you. Continue to harvest wellness and wisdom on your personal life journey and never, ever give up on your dream and vision for your life.

AFTERWORD

In the early years of my career I was privileged to work with adults with disabilities who were undertaking community based social and vocational rehabilitation training programmes. While many participants shared common interests, each person was unique in terms of their personalities, abilities and aspirations. I believed that each participant could achieve their potential if we adopted a person centered approach, which was directed toward quality of life outcomes. I undertook research on quality of life as a foundation for person centered planning, and developed a framework for rehabilitative training that was underpinned by quality of life measures. Each participant was facilitated to identify their current life satisfaction in relation to their, physical, emotional, social, spiritual, material, occupational and civic wellbeing. From this they were guided to identify the aspects of their life they wanted to address in the short term, medium term and long term.

Following this each participant developed a Personal Support Action Plan which reflected their quality of life choices, their training and development goals and the actions steps and supports required to achieve these. Meetings were held weekly with each participant to review how they were progressing with their goals and what, if anything needed to be addressed to improve their outcomes and life satisfaction. Participants also maintained a diary where they recorded what they liked doing, what worked well and what they would like to do more or less of the following week. This was a useful form of reflection and those with literacy challenges used pictures and drawings to represent their weekly reflections. The model I developed represented a move toward a whole person model where the participant is central to the training process.

Fast forward to autumn 2012 when I enrolled on health and wellness coach training with Dr Michael Arloski, Ph.D. Founder of Real Balance Global Wellness Services, Inc. I discovered that the Real Balance Wellness Mapping 360° Methodology™ developed by Dr Arloski is underpinned by the same person centred principles I had championed in my research and in my work with adults with disabilities. In wellness and health coaching the coach is a guide and ally who supports the client to identify and achieve their personal life goals. It was like coming full circle and little did I know when I undertook my research on quality of life and person centred planning that twelve years later I would be applying the same person centred principles in my work as a Health and Wellness Coach.

Our personal life journey always takes us to the place where the next aspect of our life purpose begins to unfold. We never know in advance where that place will be, but if we learn to expect the unexpected and to embrace what we face, we will enjoy the journey.

Wellness is about moving forward in your life, being open to change and new experiences, and embracing opportunities for personal fulfilment and happiness. If you embrace your personal life journey you will harvest wellness and wisdom and you will gain clarity about the direction you want to travel physically, mentally and spiritually in your life. You will become open to change and you will begin to recognise the things you can control or change, and accept that which is beyond your control. You will get excited about living and you will look forward to the unknown adventures that lie ahead.

You will come to realise that the lessons life teaches you, will strengthen your wellness foundation, unlock your fountain of wisdom, and reveal your inner truth. You will be less afraid to have a dream of a brighter future and you will not surrender this dream to fear of the unknown, or to fear of failure. Neither will you give anyone permission to trample on or dismiss your dreams. If you trip up along the way you will recognise that you have within you the resilience to pick yourself up and get back on track. You will find the courage to reach out and ask for help or support when you are struggling. You will recognise that you need the support of others to achieve your dreams and goals; therefore you will not hesitate to ask for help.

Every day you will choose to live by your inner truth, and as you do so, you will take another step toward fulfilling your life purpose, and finding inner peace and happiness. You will continue to strengthen your wellness foundation and your quality of life and life satisfaction will improve. You will understand and accept that it is your divine right to have a wellness filled life, and you will do what it takes to assert that right. You will celebrate living and you will learn to give thanks and express gratitude for the wonderful gift that is your life. As you achieve, inner peace and serenity, you will blossom like the lotus flower, in the garden of your life.

Yours in wellness

Anne Marie

BIBLIOGRAPHY

Arloski, Michael. 2007. *Wellness Coaching for Lasting Lifestyle Change.* Duluth, MN: Whole Person Associates. (2nd Ed. 2009)

Burchard, Brendan. 2014. *The Motivation Manifesto: 9 Declarations t Claim Your Personal Power.* New York. Hay House

Chodron, Pema. 2000. *When Things Fall Apart: Heart Advice for Difficult Times.* Shambhala Publications, Inc.

Frizzell, Anne Marie. "Quality of Life as a Foundation for Person Centred Planning in Social and Vocational Rehabilitation Services for Adults with Learning Disabilities". MSc diss. University College Dublin (2000)

Myss, Caroline. *1997. Anatomy of the Spirit: The Seven Stages of Power and Healing.* London. Harmony: Random House

Pink, Daniel H. 2009. *Drive: The Surprising Truth About What Motivates Us.* New York: Riverhead Books Penguin group

Ruiz-Miguel, Don. 1997. *The Four Agreements: A Guide to Personal Freedom.* California: Amber-Allen Publishing

Tolle, Eckhart. 2006. *A New Earth: Create A Better Life.* London: Penguin Books

Zinn-Kabat, Jon and Myla Kabat-Zinn. 1998. *Everyday Blessings: The Inner Work of Mindful Parenting.* New York: Hyperion

ABOUT THE AUTHOR

Anne Marie Frizzell is a Registered Nurse, a Dietary Coach and a Health and Wellness Coach. She is a member of the International Coaching Federation Irish Charter Chapter, and a Coaching Awards Finalist 2015. Anne Marie is committed to positively influencing the health and wellness of individuals and communities, by supporting them to build their Personal Wellness Foundation. She lives in Yeats County, Sligo, Ireland with her daughter Erica.

RESOURCES

www.welllifejourney.com
www.realbalance.com
www.thetappingsolution.com

Lightning Source UK Ltd.
Milton Keynes UK
UKOW04f0758301215

265513UK00001B/9/P